Sebastian Vonhoff

Microparticle Formation by Spray-Freeze-Drying

Sebastian Vonhoff

Microparticle Formation by Spray-Freeze-Drying

The Influence of Atomization Conditions on Protein Secondary and Tertiary Structure

Südwestdeutscher Verlag für Hochschulschriften

Impressum/Imprint (nur für Deutschland/ only for Germany)
Bibliografische Information der Deutschen Nationalbibliothek: Die Deutsche Nationalbibliothek verzeichnet diese Publikation in der Deutschen Nationalbibliografie; detaillierte bibliografische Daten sind im Internet über http://dnb.d-nb.de abrufbar.

Verlag: Südwestdeutscher Verlag für Hochschulschriften Aktiengesellschaft & Co. KG
Dudweiler Landstr. 99, 66123 Saarbrücken, Deutschland
Telefon +49 681 37 20 271-1, Telefax +49 681 37 20 271-0
Email: info@svh-verlag.de
Zugl.: Erlangen, FAU Erlangen-Nürnberg, Dissertation, 2010

Herstellung in Deutschland:
Schaltungsdienst Lange o.H.G., Berlin
Books on Demand GmbH, Norderstedt
Reha GmbH, Saarbrücken
Amazon Distribution GmbH, Leipzig
ISBN: 978-3-8381-1771-3

Imprint (only for USA, GB)
Bibliographic information published by the Deutsche Nationalbibliothek: The Deutsche Nationalbibliothek lists this publication in the Deutsche Nationalbibliografie; detailed bibliographic data are available in the Internet at http://dnb.d-nb.de.

Publisher: Südwestdeutscher Verlag für Hochschulschriften Aktiengesellschaft & Co. KG
Dudweiler Landstr. 99, 66123 Saarbrücken, Germany
Phone +49 681 37 20 271-1, Fax +49 681 37 20 271-0
Email: info@svh-verlag.de

Printed in the U.S.A.
Printed in the U.K. by (see last page)
ISBN: 978-3-8381-1771-3

Für meinen Vater,
der genau in diesem Moment
(immer noch) in der Apotheke steht.

Tu ne quaesieris, scire nefas, quem mihi, quem tibi
finem di dederint, Leuconoe, nec Babylonios
temptaris numeros. ut melius, quidquid erit, pati.
seu pluris hiemes seu tribuit Iuppiter ultimam,
quae nunc oppositis debilitat pumicibus mare
Tyrrhenum: sapias, vina liques, et spatio brevi
spem longam reseces. dum loquimur, fugerit invida
aetas: carpe diem quam minimum credula postero.

Horaz, Carmen 1,11

ACKNOWLEDGEMENTS

The research work presented in this thesis has been performed between June 2006 and November 2009 at the Department of Pharmaceutical Technology, University of Erlangen-Nuremberg, Erlangen, Germany.

First of all, Prof. Dr. Geoffrey Lee is gratefully acknowledged for offering me the opportunity to work in the Division of Pharmaceutics, for serving as my doctoral advisor, and for refereeing this thesis.

Many thanks go to Dr. Heiko Schiffter, for his continuous and extensive support throughout my work. You always found time for discussing arising problems with me and made the distance between Erlangen and Oxford completely insignificant. In addition, you supervised me in a cooperative and friendly way that I did not take for granted. Thank you for that and I hope we stay in contact in the years to come.

Prof. Dr. Wolfgang Frieß, Department of Pharmaceutics, University of Munich, is thanked for kindly being co-referee for this thesis.

Dr. Stefan Schneid, aka "Snütje", is kindly acknowledged for thoroughly proof-reading this work, for introducing me to "How I met your mother" - the by far greatest sitcom on the planet, and the fruitful scientific and personal discussions we had in our lab. This thesis would not have been possible without you in this form.

I would also like to thank all my present and former colleagues in the Department of Pharmaceutics. First of all Georg Straller, with whom I had the pleasure of battling for the title "sWdW". We experienced the same ups and downs during our work which made things a lot easier. Then of course Simone Reismann, whose sunny disposition was always a welcome diversion, Jakob Beirowski for lots of open-minded discussions in a wide variety of subjects, and Susanne Rutzinger for our many funny conversations. I'd also like to thank Elke Lorentzen, Peter Lassner, Eva Wulsten, Harald Pudritz, Anke Sass and Eva Meister for the friendly atmosphere and the good times at the department as well as Dr. Henning Gieseler for the good discussions we had and his clear point-of-view.

Within the department, I would first like to thank Josef Hubert for building or fixing almost anything that I came up with. You made McGyver look like an innocent school boy. Also, I will never forget our mutual trip to the Netherlands and back - all in one day without even having a working car radio. Then, Petra Neubarth for taking care of administrative things and the very nice conversations we had, Dr. Stefan Seyferth for our good talks and for handling any issues I had concerning IT and the Playstation 3, Luise Schedl for taking all of the SEM pictures presented in this work and Christiane Blaha for the fast and reliable ordering of supplies.

I'd also like to acknowledge my former students Steffi Purkl and Joachim Schäfer for the hard work they provided while working under my supervision. You have been a great help.

Finally, I want to express my gratitude to my father Hans-Jürgen, my brother Christian and my aunt Susanne for their continuous support during the last years - you made all of this possible. And last but not least, I would like to thank my girlfriend Joanna for her never-ending patience over the last months, for starting a complete new life with me, and for being a wonderful mother to our little daughter Lea. You're far from ordinary :*

PARTS OF THIS THESIS HAVE ALREADY BEEN PRESENTED OR PUBLISHED

I. Sebastian Vonhoff, Heiko Schiffter, Jamie Condliffe, Geoffrey Lee (2007). "Investigation of protein process stability during spray-freeze-drying (SFD) using FTIR and fluorescence spectroscopy." AAPS Annual Meeting. San Diego (USA).

II. Sebastian Vonhoff, Heiko Schiffter (2008). "Implementation of an FTIR calibration curve for fast and objective determination of changes in protein secondary structure." AAPS Annual Meeting. Atlanta (USA).

III. Sebastian Vonhoff, Heiko Schiffter (2008). "Influence of nozzle-type and atomization conditions on protein secondary and tertiary structure during spray-freeze-drying." AAPS Annual Meeting. Atlanta (USA).

IV. Sebastian Vonhoff, Jamie Condliffe, Heiko Schiffter (2009). "Implementation of an FTIR calibration curve for fast and objective determination of changes in protein secondary structure during formulation development." Journal of Pharmaceutical and Biopharmaceutical Analysis 51(1): 39-45

List of abbreviations

ΔT	Temperature difference
ε_λ	Absorptivity constant
λ	Wavelength
A_λ	Absorbance at given wavelength
a-CT	α-chymotrypsin
API	Active pharmaceutical ingredient
AU	Arbitrary unit
b	Pathlength
c	Concentration
CD	Circular dichroism
CLS	Classic least squares
CMC	Critical micelle concentration
d_v	Mean volume diameter
$d_{v,50}$	Median of volume diameters
EMEA	European medicines agency
FD	Freeze-drying
FDA	Food and drug administration
Fe	Ammonium iron(II) sulfate hexahydrate
FTIR	Fourier transform infrared spectroscopy
HSA	Human serum albumin
IEP	Isoelectric point

ILS	Inverse least squares
IR	Infrared
K_λ	Proportionality factor at given wavelength
KI	Potassium iodide
LN_2	Liquid nitrogen
MRDP	Major R_x drug portfolio
PLS	Partial least squares
PRESS	Predicted residual error sum of squares
r	Correlation coefficient
R^2	Coefficient of determination
Re	Reynolds number
rh	Relative humidity
RMSE	Root mean square error
R_x	Available on prescription
sdv	standard deviation
SEM	Scanning electron microscopy
SFD or SFV/L	Spray-freeze-drying into vapor over liquid
SSA	Specific surface area
SVD	Singular value decomposition
T	Transpose
T_g	Glass transition temperature
T_g'	Glass transition temperature of the maximum concentrated solute
T_m	Melting temperature
TA	Terephthalic acid

We	Weber number

Table of contents

1. Introduction

Biopharmaceuticals, also known as biologics, present a comparably new class of drug substances including rather complex API's such as hormones, cytokines, clotting factors, monoclonal antibodies or enzymes [Dudzinski et al. 2008]. Many biologics have already been approved by FDA and EMEA, offering high therapeutic potential for treatment of serious illnesses such as rheumatoid arthritis (Enbrel®), breast cancer (Herceptin®), multiple sclerosis (Humira®) or anemia (Epogen®) [Engelberg et al. 2009]. From the industry's point of view economic prospects concerning biologics for the coming years are also very promising. According to a recent market analysis by Goodman [2009], the average share of biologics in the major R_x drug portfolios (MRDP) of the 14 largest capitalization pharmaceutical companies is expected to increase from 26% in 2008 to 40% in 2013. As drugs included in the MRDP are predicted to achieve at least US$ 500 million in annual sales, this development will have severe impact on other pharmaceutical companies and their product pipelines as well. On the other hand, the contribution from small-molecule drugs to portfolio revenue is expected to stagnate or decrease mostly due to patent expirations of older blockbuster drugs.

Until now, the market is mostly protected from generic biologics – the so-called biosimilars. Although the FDA currently evaluates an abbreviated approval pathway, it seems unlikely that hurdles, such as expensive immunogenicity studies and clinical trials, could be completely avoided [Engelberg et al. 2009]. This guarantees recovery of the research and development costs as well as high revenues for new biological drugs in the following years.

The manufacturing of protein pharmaceuticals is a very complicated process which generates high costs during their development. Prior to designing an adept administration scheme, the API itself either has to be extracted from tissue or generated from bacterial or mammalian expression systems, such as recombinant proteins. The interested reader is referred to literature for an in-depth description of the manufacturing of recombinant proteins and peptides [Makrides 1996; Graumann et al. 2006]. Depending on the intended way of administration, the active agent can be processed in various ways and combined with necessary excipients, thus forming the final drug product. In spite of various improvements in drug delivery by nano- and microparticulate systems, oral bioavailability is still limited due to intestinal membrane permeability, molecule size, intestinal and hepatic metabolism and solubility [Malik et al. 2007]. Therefore, protein pharmaceuticals are most commonly applied the parenteral way.

Parenteral protein formulations, however, often suffer from inferior stability during long-term storage – especially in the liquid state (see chapter 2.2.2). Freeze-drying or lyophilization has become the method of choice for stabilizing those labile APIs. By removing water as the main partner during degradation reactions, shelf-life can be drastically increased while transportation and storage issues are reduced [Vonhoff 2009]. The lyophilized cake can be reconstituted again prior to its administration and is then immediately ready for use. However, the removal of water itself as well as other stress factors like cold denaturation, potential pH shifts etc. can damage the protein during freeze-drying, making it sometimes hard to find ideal formulation and process conditions [Costantino et al. 2004].

There are ways of parenteral drug delivery, such as needle-free injection or systemic inhalation therapy, that offer obvious advantages over conventional invasive administration via needle and syringe [Burkoth et al. 1999; Siekmeier et al. 2008]. Compliance is enhanced by the absence of needles, while applicability is improved by using the powder without prior reconstitution. Additionally, the danger of transmitting serious infections, such as hepatitis B and C or HIV, through needle-stick injuries can be ruled out making both methods very safe. One prominent, but unsuccessful example for systemic drug delivery by powder inhalation was Pfizer's Exubera® (see Fig. 1.1). It was withdrawn from the market in October 2007 after it failed to achieve an acceptable market share. Apart from side effects like coughing, dry mouth or shortness of breath, the inhaler suffered from avoidable design failures: The smallest blister pack contained an equivalent of 3U insulin which made it hard to achieve accurate dosage control. Furthermore, the Exubera® inhaler had the size of a 200 mL water glass when closed which actually doubled if opened for inhalation [Siekmeier et al. 2008]. Hence, Exubera® clearly performed below its potential and sadly ended the development of analogous products as well. Today, only Mannkind is working on a phase III trial for inhaled insulin (Technosphere®).

For the above mentioned applications, a fine powder with defined properties is needed instead of a coherent cake as produced by regular freeze-drying. Hence, different processing technologies become necessary for the manufacturing of the final drug products. Spray-drying (SD) is probably by far the most popular method for the generation of microparticles, while spray-freeze-drying (SFD) presents a newer promising alternative.

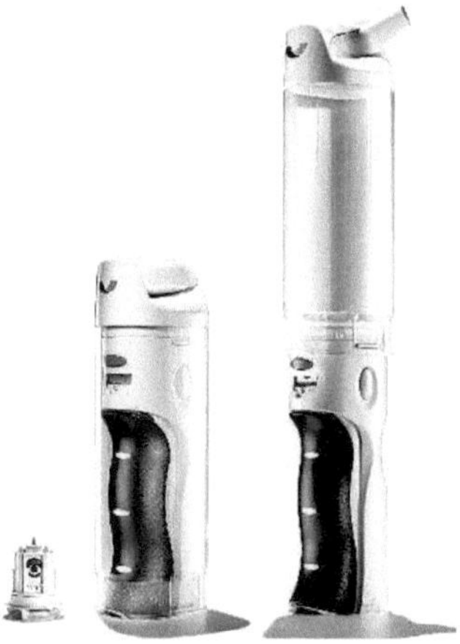

Fig. 1.1: Picture of the Exubera® inhalation device in the closed (left) and opened state (right).

Maa et al. [1999] compared both techniques for the preparation of fine aerosol particles suitable for inhalation. They found out that SD is the faster and easier process as it is already well-established, and refined benchtop spray-dryers are commercially available. Spray-freeze-drying, on the other hand, was able to deliver particles at a higher yield (>95%) with superior aerosol performance, thus making SFD potentially the more economical process for expensive formulations. They also stated that SFD might exhibit the more stressful processing steps than spray-drying, making it necessary to further investigate the influence of SFD on labile APIs. Even though numerous evaluations concerning the individual processing steps of SFD have been published [Costantino et al. 2000; Costantino et al. 2002; Sonner et al. 2002; Yu et al. 2006], no systematic investigation has been performed in regard to different atomization conditions and their effect on protein stability. The choice of nozzle type (two-fluid or ultrasound nozzle) can have noticeable influence on various parameters of the spraying step, such as droplet size, temperature stress or cavitation effects. By applying disadvantageous atomization conditions, labile APIs could already be damaged during this first unit operation, thus reducing the feasibility of the whole process.

One technique of analysis that has been widely used for determining protein stability during FD is FTIR spectroscopy. It offers the unique ability to analyze samples in the solid and liquid state which is advantageous for lyophilization. Furthermore, effects, such as unfolding and aggregation during freeze-drying are known to directly correlate with protein secondary and tertiary structure [Carpenter et al. 1998]. Finally, prolonged storage stability has been connected to the preservation of protein secondary structure during lyophilization [Rey et al. 2004; Chang et al. 2005]. Therefore,

FTIR spectroscopy can also provide valuable information concerning the level of protein stress during the individual processing steps of SFD. As the evaluation of protein FTIR spectra can be rather subjective (see chapter 3.2) some reviews have doubted the validity of FTIR analysis [Haris et al. 1992; Jackson et al. 1995]. Hence, great care must be taken when choosing an evaluation method in order to obtain objective and reproducible results.

In this thesis the generation of protein loaded microparticles by SFD is evaluated. Emphasis lies on protein secondary structure and its dependency on varying atomization conditions. Therefore, a new and objective quantification algorithm for FTIR analysis is created during a first set of experiments. Then, this evaluation method is used to determine damage to protein secondary structure during SFD at different atomization conditions in a second series of experiments. Stability evaluations also include protein tertiary structure by fluorescence spectroscopy as well as overall enzyme activity by UV/Vis spectroscopic assay, where possible. This permits a comprehensive view on the stability of α-chymotrypsin and human serum albumin, which are both used as model proteins in the SFD experiments in this work. Additionally, temperature and cavitation measurements from different nozzle types give insight into possible stress factors for labile APIs during ultrasound atomization. In a last series of experiments, information gained throughout the previous chapters is used for finding appropriate stabilizing excipients for α-chymotrypsin during SFD at different experimental setups. In summary, the findings in this work should enhance the understanding of this rather new particle engineering process and facilitate the creation of stable protein formulation for spray-freeze-drying.

2. Spray-freeze-drying of proteins

2.1 Overview of spray-freeze-drying methods

Spray-freeze-drying is a rather new technology for the generation of distinct spherical particles. In general, a liquid feed solution or suspension is atomized above or within a container filled with a cryogenic liquid or cryogenic gas. The fine droplets of the spray are almost instantly frozen and turned into distinct ice particles that are suspended within the cryogen. Liquid nitrogen (LN_2) is most commonly used for this purpose, as it is chemically inert, not flammable and enables very low temperatures (-195.8°C). In addition, it is toxicological harmless and therefore very well suited for the requirements of SFD [Linde 2008]. Other coolants, such as liquid propane or isopentane, which show differences in boiling point as well as heat capacity, have also been utilized [Engstrom et al. 2007; Gieseler et al. 2009]. However, those cryogens offer an increased risk potential because they are flammable and can form explosive mixtures with oxygen during the SFD process.

Drying of the frozen particles is performed after the cryogen has been boiled off by a classic lyophilization cycle at low temperature and pressure. Temperatures during the primary drying step usually lie at -15°C or even below if the T_g' of some stabilizers make it necessary [Tang et al. 2004]. During secondary drying, shelf temperatures can be increased up to +50°C. Still, protein temperature stress is comparably low as it is already in a relatively dry state [Tang et al. 2004]. In result, protein damage due to heat denaturation can be avoided by SFD.

As stated above, the fine droplets after atomization are instantly frozen upon contact with the cryogen. If the atomized solution contains a sufficiently high solid content, the shape of the droplets is preserved, even after the removal of ice during lyophilization. Thus, particles size distribution of the final product can be controlled by atomizing the liquid feed at the desired droplet diameters [Maa et al. 2000]. The resulting product usually exhibits a highly porous structure and very large specific surface area which are caused by the rapid freezing. That's why spray-freeze-drying can be employed for enhancing the solubility of otherwise poorly water-soluble drugs [Hu et al. 2002]. Gieseler [2009] found that drying behavior of the microparticles inside freeze-drying vials is different compared to classic lyophilization. Drying rate is limited by the poor heat transfer through the large interparticular voids. However, no in-depth investigation of the drying kinetics of SFD particles has been published yet.

Spray-freezing has been successfully employed, amongst others, for generating particles with defined particle sizes usable for e.g. pulmonary delivery of anti-IgE monoclonal antibodies or epidermal powder immunization by vaccines [Abdul-Fattah et al. 2007]. Depending on the experimental setup, one usually discerns between atmospheric spray-freeze-drying (ASFD), spray-freezing into vapor over liquid (SFV/L or SFD) and spray-freezing into liquid (SFL).

2.1.1 Atmospheric spray-freeze-drying

During atmospheric spray-freeze-drying, a solution or suspension containing the API is atomized inside a spray tower and instantly frozen by a cryogen. The ice is subsequently removed by sublimation under atmospheric pressure, while the necessary heat energy is provided by convection through the fluidizing air flow. The corresponding experimental setup was first described by Leuenberger [1987] and can either use a cold air stream (-60°C) or a cooling medium consisting of solid particles, such as pulverized dry ice. Before entering the spraying tower, the air stream is desiccated by a refrigerator and a condenser. Temperatures are kept right below the eutectic temperature or the glass transition temperature of the solution to prevent the frozen particles from collapse. This way, the air is capable of taking up humidity corresponding to the modified h,x-diagram by sublimation, thus drying the frozen particles. An air filter is used to keep the product inside the spray tower during the whole procedure. Due to the high air velocity, the particles are conveyed towards the air filter and can be collected thereof, after the process is completed [Leuenberger 2002]. The apparatus has recently been further enhanced by Wang et al. [2006]. By adding several air outlets to the side walls, they could reduce deposition of the frozen particles on the side walls, thereby increasing yield of the final product.

Atmospheric spray-freeze-drying has been previously employed for the production of fine, free flowing powders at shorter drying times than conventional freeze-drying [Wang et al. 2006]. Secondary structure of e.g. BSA was completely maintained during the process, indicating that it could be suitable for other labile APIs as well. However, this technique has been rarely used in the past for the generation of protein loaded particles. Therefore, only little data is available for assessing the effects of this method on those labile biopharmaceuticals.

2.1.2 Spray-freezing into liquid

In spray-freezing into liquid, the formulation containing the active pharmaceutical ingredient (API) is forwarded by a HPLC pump through a valve to an insulated nozzle. The nozzle usually consists of a capillary made from polyetheretherketone (PEEK) that is immersed into a cryogen. Isolation is especially important as the small capillary tends to freeze rapidly which results in clogging of the nozzle. [Williams 2005]. SFL is derived in part from the PCA (Precipitation with Compressed Fluid Antisolvent) process. Atomization is performed by utilizing liquid-liquid impingement of a feed solution through a nozzle that is submerged into a fluid cryogen. The liquid feed is forwarded at high velocity through a fine orifice (inner diameter. 63.5 – 125 μm) and experiences strong friction while passing through the coolant. This leads to intense atomization of the liquid jet into micronized droplets. Engstrom et al. [2008] investigated the dependency of the jet breakup on the density and viscosity of different cryogens by calculating the corresponding Weber (*We*) and Reynolds (*Re*) numbers. The found that for spraying into LN_2 ($We = 2.0 \times 10^3$) and isopentane ($We = 2.8 \times 10^3$), the Weber numbers were two order of magnitudes higher than for spraying into gaseous nitrogen ($We = 11$) which led to no atomization. The Rayleigh numbers, on the other hand, remained unaltered because liquid feed rate was not changed during these experiments. Therefore, atomization is only possible if sufficient friction is provided by the cryogen.

The fine droplets freeze almost instantly resulting in extremely porous (sub)micron particles. Protein denaturation during the atomization step is unlikely as the time frame for adsorbing to the droplet surface is very limited [Yu et al. 2006]. Due to the very rapid freezing no phase separation can be observed and the API is homogenously dispersed within the excipient matrix. However, Engstrom et al. [2007] found out that cooling rates for SFL were strongly reduced during the processing of concentrated solutions (> 50 mg/mL). The low heat of vaporization of LN_2 led to an augmented Leidenfrost effect, thereby forming an insulating gaseous layer around the droplets. Still, freezing rates are very rapid compared to conventional lyophilization. After the atomization step is completed, the frozen particles can be collected on a sieve and transferred into a freeze-dryer for lyophilization. During this step any ice is being removed, thus leading to the final product.

Rogers et al. [2002] investigated the incorporation of donazol into hydroxypropyl-β-cyclodextrin by SFL. Donazol was homogeneously dispersed within the excipient matrix resulting in a completely amorphous product. Additionally, the API could be dissolved very quickly and showed an increased in vivo bioavailability in mouse model due to its high specific surface area [Rogers et al. 2003; Purvis et al. 2006]. The process has also been successfully adapted to proteins: Yu et al. [2002]

manufactured insulin microparticles by SFL that showed a low bulk density, high specific surface area, narrow particle size distribution and no loss in stability determined by absence of covalent dimer in SEC-HPLC. In another study, Yu et al. [2004] used SFL to generate BSA microparticles from comparably low concentrated solutions, that exhibited high protein stability. Monomer loss detected by SEC-HPLC was below 1% while native secondary structure was changed by roughly 6% from α-helix into β-sheet at most. Finally, Engstrom et al. [2007] were able to produce microparticles from solutions containing 0.25 mg/mL LDH and 30 mg/mL or 100 mg/mL trehalose, that showed nearly complete preservation of enzyme activity.

2.1.3 Spray-freezing into vapor over liquid

The main difference between SFL and SFD lies within the atomization step. In SFL a PEEK capillary that is immerged into the cryogen serves as a one-fluid nozzle requiring high pressures. In SFD, the point of spraying is positioned a few centimeters above the surface of the cryogen [Sonner 2002; Rochelle 2005]. The liquid feed is forwarded by a suitable pump, and atomized into fine droplets by either ultrasound oscillation (ultrasonic nozzles) or an atomizing air flow (two-fluid nozzles) [Maa et al. 1999; Maa et al. 2004]. During their descent through the cold vapor phase, the droplets begin to freeze and solidify completely upon contact with the cryogen [Yu et al. 2006]. Size distribution of the frozen particles can easily be controlled by nozzle parameters. For ultrasound nozzles, higher frequencies lead to smaller droplet diameters while droplet size from two-fluid nozzles is dependent on liquid feed rate and atomizing air-flow. Smaller particles lead to faster freezing rates and thus to the generation of smaller ice crystals which increases the SSA [Engstrom et al. 2007]. The final product can be transformed into nanoparticles by subsequent ultrasound sonication if the porosity is high enough [Costantino et al. 2000]. Other studies showed that SFD is adept for creating microparticles with increased density and remarkable physical stability if high solid contents are used. This makes SFD a highly versatile process for particle generation [Maa et al. 2004].

Van Drooge et al. [2005] showed that SFD is a suitable process for incorporating THC in inulin glass matrices, resulting in powders with a particle size appropriate for inhalation. Maa et al. [1999] also demonstrated that SFD is a feasible way for manufacturing protein powders suitable for pulmonary delivery. By combining rhDNase and anti-IgE antibodies with different carbohydrate excipients, they were able to generate powders with a high fine particle fraction that showed very good aerosol performance. In other studies, Maa et al. [2003; 2004] prepared influenza and hepatitis

B vaccine dry powder formulations by SFD, suitable for epidermal powder immunization. The particles exhibited high density while still preserving stability, potency and immunogenicity.

However, the prolonged time frame between atomization and complete freezing can lead to adverse effects: First, the unfrozen droplets can merge with each other while passing through the vapor phase resulting in a broad and inhomogeneous particle size distribution [Hu et al. 2004]. Second, studies showed higher protein damage during SFD in comparison to SFL with protein adsorption at the air/liquid interface [Costantino et al. 2000; Yu et al. 2006]. These findings were supported by Webb et al. [2002], who determined an elevated nitrogen amount on the surface of SFD particles by electron spectroscopy for chemical analysis (ESCA). Nitrogen was present only in the investigated protein, and therefore could be used as marker for quantifying surface adsorption tendencies. Hence, some proteins are able to unfold at the droplet surface, in spite of the very limited time frame for adsorption and the fast freezing rates. After the spraying step is completed, the frozen particles are collected and then transferred onto the pre-cooled shelves of a freeze-dryer. From that point on, any further processing is equal to the SFL process described in chapter 2.1.2.

The choice between SFL and SFD as particle manufacturing process should be made depending on the intended properties of the final product. SFL has shown to inflict less damage to labile APIs and to be very well suited for the generation of (sub)micron particles. However, it lacks the flexibility of SFD where particle size and properties can be easily changed by altering formulation properties or atomization conditions. In addition, SFD shows improved feasibility over SFL as its equipment standards are generally lower. In SFL, high liquid pressure and feed rates are applied to achieve atomization, and the nozzle is immersed directly into LN_2. This makes HPLC pump systems as well as special insulation of the PEEK capillary necessary.

As can be seen in the above paragraphs, information on the spray-freeze-drying process is rather limited. Most of the work has been performed by only few authors, which suggests that investigations are not comprehensive. Especially the atomization step, being the main difference in protein stress between SFD and SFL, has so far only been thoroughly analyzed for two-fluid nozzles by Costantino et al. [2000]. Hence, a detailed evaluation of the influence of different atomization conditions on protein stability during SFD is a promising approach for gaining further insight into this rather new particle manufacturing process.

2.2 Proteins

Proteins fulfill a wide variety of different tasks inside the human body. Amongst others, they catalyze reactions, transport other molecules, are part of the immune defense, translate nerve impulses and control growth of the body [Stryer et al. 2008]. Due to their complex structure, proteins often have the disadvantage of limited stability (especially in the liquid state) and applicability (mostly as parenteral dosage forms). Therefore, much work has been put into developing stable protein formulations in the past, with plenty of advises available in the literature concerning drying techniques, additives, degradation pathways, etc [Izutsu et al. 2004; Chang et al. 2005; Abdul-Fattah et al. 2008].

2.2.1 Protein structure

Primary structure

The most basic structural feature of a protein is its primary structure. It consists of a linear strand of L-amino acids that are covalently connected by a peptide bond. One can discern between a protein's main chain – the so-called protein backbone – and the side chains that vary dependent on the amino acids incorporated. Short chains of amino acids are usually referred to as peptides or oligopeptides. Titin with its 27000 amino acids is the largest known protein in the human body and has a weight of 3000 kDa. The sequence of the individual monomers is unique to one specific protein [Stryer et al. 2008].

Secondary structure

The primary structure of a protein exhibits a certain degree of flexibility. This makes it possible to arrange the amino acids in a number of different conformations. These secondary structures are stabilized by intramolecular hydrogen bonds between the CO and NH groups of the amide functions [Stryer et al. 2008]. Corey [1951] and Pauling [1951] first postulated the existence of α-helix and β-sheet structure by analyzing the sterically possible foldings of peptides. Later, conformations like β-turn and Ω-loop were added as well. The α-helix is formed by a twisted protein backbone with the side-chains of the individual amino acids oriented towards the outside. It is usually arranged right handed in proteins with 3.6 monomers necessary for one complete turn [Stryer et al. 2008]. In β-sheets, the peptide strand is extended which leads to a completely different overall shape. The distances between the peptide bonds are longer (0.35 nm vs. 0.15 nm in α-helix) which leads to weaker dipole interactions. Neighboring β-sheet strands can be oriented in the same (parallel) or in the opposite direction (antiparallel) depending on the β-turns and Ω-loops available [Stryer et al. 2008].

Tertiary structure

The individual structural features described in the above paragraph can also be arranged in various ways. In an aqueous system the protein tries to bury its hydrophobic side-chains in the interior while the hydrophilic residues can be found at the outside. This leads to the formation of a protein's tertiary structure. The tertiary structure of an enzyme can be essential for its activity as it enables amino acid side-chains, located at different positions within the primary structure, to interact with each other. This way, active centers like the "catalytic triad" described in chapter 4.1 become possible [Stryer et al. 2008]. An in-depth review of protein folding patterns has been presented by [Chothia et al. 1990]

Protein quaternary structure

Finally, a protein can also consist of more than just one polypeptide strand. Different subunits can associate thus forming the active state of the protein [Stryer et al. 2008].

Protein secondary and tertiary structure both are of special interest when investigating the generation of protein loaded particles by SFD. Processing steps such as atomization or rapid freezing can lead to denaturation of the protein [Costantino et al. 2000]. As can be seen in section 2.2.3, denaturation is directly linked to a loss in native protein folding and therefore can be monitored by quantifying protein secondary and tertiary structure. Additionally, water removal during the lyophilization step is critical for the SFD process, as it potentially disturbs essential hydrogen bonds between the protein and surrounding water molecules [Pikal-Cleland et al. 2001]. This can lead to changes in protein secondary structure as well. Finally, storage stability is generally considered to increase with preservation of native protein secondary structure [Carpenter et al. 1998]. Hence, evaluation of changes to secondary and tertiary structure can be valuable tools to quantify possible protein stress factors during SFD.

2.2.2 Chemical degradation pathways

The complex structural features described in chapter 2.2.1 are the main cause for the many possible degradation pathways of proteins. It is common to discern between chemical and physical instabilities. Any changes incorporating bond formation or cleavage yielding a new chemical entity are referred to as chemical instabilities. Physical instabilities, on the other hand, correspond to changes in higher order structures (secondary structure or higher) [Manning et al. 1989]. As chemical degradation pathways were not investigated in this thesis, they are only briefly described in Table 2.1.

Table 2.1: Overview of different chemical degradation pathways [Manning et al. 1989].

Chemical instability	Meaning
Deamidation	The amide function of a glutamine or asparagine side chain can be hydrolyzed, thus forming a free carboxylic acid.
Oxidation	Oxidation of the amino acid side chains of tryptophan, methionine or cysteine by air.
Hydrolysis	Hydrolysis of the aspartyl peptide bond.
Disulfide exchange	Interchange of existing disulfide bonds.
Racemization	Change of the configuration of chiral amino acids.
β-Elimination	Part of the side chain of e.g. lysine or phenylalanine can be eliminated.

2.2.3 Physical degradation pathways

Denaturation and aggregation

Denaturation refers to alteration of the global fold of a protein thereby affecting its tertiary and (most of the time) secondary structures. While irreversible unfolding is permanent, reversible unfolding can be undone by altering certain properties of a protein preparation, such as temperature or pH [Manning et al. 1989]. When aggregation reaches a certain threshold, precipitates become visible by the naked eye. Therefore, precipitation is the macroscopic equivalent of aggregation. Usually, unfolding in aqueous solution is thought to be a cooperative transition between the native (N) and the unfolded (U) state (Equation 2.1).

Equation 2.1 $$N \leftrightarrow U$$

The temperature or conditions at which 50% of protein molecules unfold is called the melting temperature (T_m) and lies mostly between 40 – 80°C [Wang 1999].

For lyophilization, the interrelation between the different protein foldings becomes more complex. During the freezing step, the native conformation may be preserved, resulting in and undamaged frozen protein. In the presence of adept stabilizers, the subsequent removal of water does not lead to denaturation and gives the native dry state which can be reconstituted again by the addition of water. Still, there are many possible pathways for the protein to unfold, either during the freezing step, the removal of water or during reconstitution of the lyophilized cake [Prestrelski et al. 1993].

The driving force behind protein aggregation is minimization of thermodynamically unfavorable interactions between solvent and exposed hydrophobic residues after unfolding. Aggregation can be induced by chemical as well as physical triggers and may at last lead to precipitation [Wang 1999]. The unfolded state is often insoluble and favors aggregation. Therefore Equation 2.1 can be modified into Equation 2.2.

Equation 2.2 $$N \leftrightarrow U \rightarrow A$$

Still, one must keep in mind that aggregation can also emerge from a partially unfolded state. This means that a protein does not need to unfold completely before aggregation [Vermeer et al. 2000]. For example, the total amount of energy, that is necessary to transform rhIFN-γ from its native state into its completely unfolded state, is rather high. However, the protein can already form aggregates from a transition state. The energy difference between the native and the transition state is rather low which facilitates aggregation. From the transition state, the protein can form dimeric aggregates or aggregates consisting of various monomers. The addition of cosolutes is known to influence the amount of energy that is necessary for the protein to unfold. Sucrose, for example, elevates the free energy, that is necessary to reach the unfolded or transition state, while guanidine lowers the energy which corresponds to stabilization and destabilization, respectively [Chi et al. 2003].

Surface adsorption:

As proteins exhibit an amphiphilic character they are prone to adsorb to interfaces which in effect can lead to denaturation as well. Insulin for example has been reported to adsorb to surfaces of delivery pumps, glass and plastic containers and to the inside of intravenous bags [Manning et al. 1989].

Spray-freeze-drying exhibits an even higher potential for destabilizing protein preparations than lyophilization alone due to its additional spraying step: High energy input during atomization of the solution could increase temperatures, thus leading to protein denaturation (see chapter 7). In addition, the atomization step drastically enlarges the air/liquid interface, and thereby can promote protein adsorption [Costantino et al. 2000; Webb et al. 2002]. The above described freezing and drying stress is nevertheless present in SFD, potentially leading to further protein denaturation. Therefore, stabilization of the protein preparation by the addition of proper excipients can become necessary.

2.2.4 Stabilization in the liquid state

The stability of proteins in the liquid state is known to be dependent on numerous factors, such as temperature, pH, salt type, salt concentration, preservatives, surfactants and cosolutes [Chi et al. 2003]. By adding adequate excipients to the formulation, protein stability can be greatly increased. Generally, the same mechanisms that are responsible for solute-induced protein stabilization in aqueous solutions are effective during the freezing step (hence the name "cryoprotectants"). The mechanism can be explained by the preferential interaction and exclusion theory of Timasheff [2002]. Protein stabilizers such as polyols are preferentially excluded from the surface of the protein and the degree of exclusion is proportional to the surface exposed to the solvent. With increase in surface area during denaturation, exclusion of the excipient increases as well resulting in an energetically unfavorable state [Chi et al. 2003]. Surfactants, on the other hand, competitively inhibit protein adsorption to interfaces and therefore can be employed for stabilization during the spraying and freezing steps [Maa et al. 1998].

Prediction of the stability of high concentrated protein solutions is complicated. Generally one must discern between conformational stability (e.g. secondary and tertiary structure) and colloidal stability (e.g. resistance to denaturation and aggregation) [Guo 2006]. An increase in protein concentration should have a positive effect on conformational stability as proteins – just like other cosolutes – are preferentially excluded from each other's surface. At the same time colloidal stability decreases as protein-protein interactions become more likely [Minton 2000]. According to Guo [2006], the effects of using high concentrated solutions are dependent on the investigated protein and therefore cannot be generalized.

2.2.5 Stabilization in the solid state

The native conformation of a protein strongly depends on the interaction of the backbone and its side chains with water molecules. Therefore, dehydration can lead to severe perturbations of higher structures finally resulting in protein denaturation [Rupley et al. 1991]. Stabilization of proteins in the solid state is usually explained by two models. The first one is the glass dynamics hypothesis: A good stabilizer forms a rigid, inert matrix in which the protein is molecularly dispersed. Due to the reduced mobility any bimolecular reactions as well as other degradation pathways are greatly slowed down. Hence, stabilization is performed by a kinetic approach, and protein stability should correlate with molecular mobility within the matrix [Chang et al. 2005]. The quality of stabilization is often quantified in regard to the T_g value of the final product or the relaxation time constant of the amorphous matrix [Shamblin et al. 2000]. The second model is called the water substitute hypothesis. It states that a stabilizer (like sugars or other polyols) can form hydrogen bonds with the protein, thereby replacing water molecules that were available in the dissolved state. This means that denaturation is inhibited thermodynamically during the drying process by increasing the free energy of unfolding, which leads to increased stability in the solid state [Prestrelski et al. 1993]. Due to their stabilizing effect during lyophilization, excipients exhibiting the above mentioned characteristics are also referred to as "lyoprotectants".

3. FTIR spectroscopy

3.1 Basic principles and instrumentation

IR spectroscopy is a relatively old technique that has been employed for a wide variety of analytical purposes [Chalmers et al. 2001]. Elliot [1950] discovered that a correlation exists between the frequency of the amide I and II absorption bands and the secondary structure of a protein determined by X-ray diffraction. However, IR spectrometers at that time were not powerful enough for delivering a comprehensive view on secondary structure. With the breakthrough of Fourier-transform infrared spectroscopy, signal quality improved remarkably which led to an increase in informational content on protein secondary structures. Even today, FTIR equipment for protein analysis is still being improved. The Proteus transmission cell (Thermo Scientific, Waltham, USA) or the Hyperion FTIR microscope (Bruker Optics, Ettlingen, Germany) are only two examples for recent enhancements in FTIR analysis.

IR absorption is caused by the interaction of electromagnetic radiation with molecular vibrations. If the frequencies of light and vibration concur, the electromagnetic wave will amplify the oscillation of a molecule [Barth et al. 2002]. Although the number of possible vibrations grows with increasing molecule size, complexity of the spectra is reduced by the fact that not all vibrations can be resolved in the liquid state. Additionally, vibrations can only be detected if a change in dipole moment is involved which further simplifies the spectrum [van der Weert et al. 2005].

The biggest advantage of FTIR over conventional IR spectroscopy is that it employs the full IR spectrum at once instead of performing a wavelength separation by a slit. This leads to several advantages [Mauerer 2006]:

- *Multiplex advantage (Fellgett advantage)*

  Time is being reduced for acquiring a certain signal-to-noise ratio in comparison to a dispersive apparatus.
- *Throughput advantage (Jacquinot advantage)*

  The entire range and amount of IR radiation is continuously used leading to a better signal-to noise ratio.

- *Conne's advantage*

  The incorporation of a laser increases spectral detection as the position of the mirror can be determined very precisely.

The spectrometer uses an interferometer equipped with a beam splitter that divides the incident IR radiation into two beams. Both are reflected by one moving and one fixated mirror respectively (Fig. 3.1a), then reunited again and sent through the sample towards the detector. Dependent on the position of the moving mirror, the interferences can be constructive or destructive, leading to a rather complex interferogram (Fig. 3.1b). The relation between signal intensity and mirror position can be described by Equation 3.1.

Equation 3.1 $$I(x) = \int_0^\infty I(x,\bar{v})\,d\bar{v} = \frac{1}{2}\int_0^\infty I(\bar{v})[1+\cos(2\pi\bar{v}x)]d\bar{v}$$

where x is the way of the mirror and $\bar{v}$ is the wavenumber ($1/\lambda$).

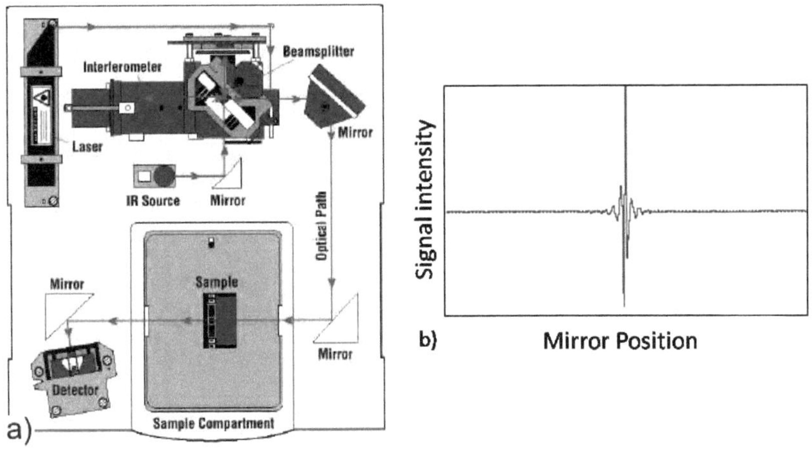

Fig. 3.1: a) Schematics of a FTIR spectroscope showing the function of the interferometer and the beam splitter (Picture taken from Mauerer [2006]) b) Typical interferogram.

By performing a Fourier transform, Equation 3.1 can be transformed from a position dependent into a wavenumber dependent formula (Equation 3.2), thus revealing the final spectrum.

Equation 3.2 $$I(\overline{v}) = \int_0^{\infty} I(x,\overline{v})dx$$

As the number of data points and the maximum pathlength of the two mirrors are finite, the infinite integral in Equation 3.1 becomes finite as well which complicates the calculation of the Fourier transform. These problems can be overcome by approximations known as Fast Fourier transforms. Further possible adjustments can be performed by a weighting function ("apodization") and by adding additional zeros in the interferogram ("zero-filling"). However, the effects of both techniques on protein spectra are either unsure or unnecessary and therefore should be used with caution [van der Weert et al. 2005].

Apart from the interferometer, a FTIR spectroscope consists of an IR source, a laser, a sample chamber and a detector. The laser is used for determining the exact position of the moving mirror which increases resolution. Additionally, the laser is also used as trigger for data acquisition. Two types of detectors are being used for FTIR spectroscopy – a deuterated triglycine sulfate (dTGS) and a mercury-cadmium-telluride (MCT) detector. The latter has a shorter response time than the dTGS detector which allows faster spectrum recording. On the downside, the MCT shows a smaller linear range and must be cooled with LN_2 which slightly reduces its applicability.

3.2 Evaluation methods and experimental considerations

Depending on recording conditions and the applied evaluation method, quantification of protein secondary structure by FTIR spectroscopy can be prone to failure. As observable in the following paragraphs, different approaches have been undertaken in the past to quantify secondary structures and their changes, each one of them offering advantages and disadvantages. Correct information can only be obtained by recording spectra at optimal experimental conditions and by choosing an objective evaluation method suited for the task at hand.

The peptide bonds of the protein give rise to three major signals within the FTIR absorbance spectrum, referred to as the amide I, II and III band (Fig. 3.2). The amide I band (1700 cm^{-1}-1600 cm^{-1}) is used by most authors for the determination of secondary structure as it is built up by few molecule vibrations with plenty of information available in literature [Susi et al. 1985; Dong et al. 1995; Carpenter et al. 1998]. The amide II band (1600 cm^{-1}-1500 cm^{-1}) is mostly employed for evaluating the accessibility of the protein backbone by H-D exchange [Haris et al. 1990; Wu 2001], while the amide III band (1330 cm^{-1}-1220 cm^{-1}) is only seldom utilized for structural evaluation due to its weak intensity and complex composition [Costantino et al. 1995].

Two important factors that must be considered prior to quantifying secondary structure using the amide I band are the residual water vapor and the subtraction of the background spectrum from the recorded protein sample.

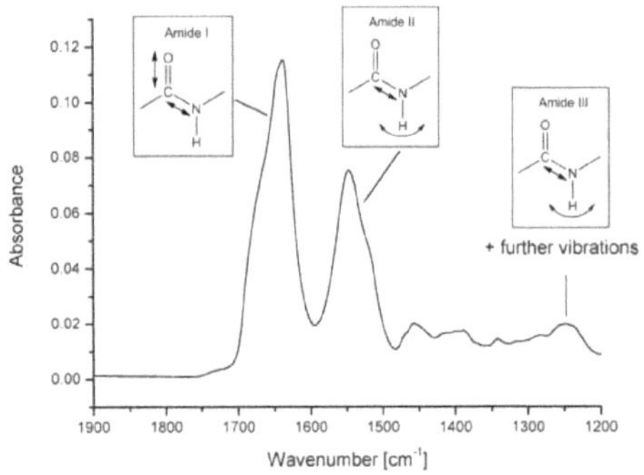

Fig. 3.2: Pure protein spectrum of a-CT showing its three amide bands and the underlying vibrations [Vonhoff 2009].

Water absorbs in the very same region as the amide I band which can lead to complications. If the relative humidity (rh) within the measurement chamber changes between background and sample recording, sharp peaks assigned to water vapor are visible in the subtraction spectrum. This makes it impossible to reliably quantify secondary structure content, especially if second derivative or Fourier self-deconvolution are applied [Jackson et al. 1995].

Subtraction of the background spectrum is critical, especially if excipients have been added for stabilization of the protein. As can be seen in Fig. 3.3, spectra can be weighed differently during subtraction by applying a multiplication factor. This leads to the danger of over- and undersubtracting individual components if incorrect values are chosen (compare the regions between 1700 cm^{-1} and 1600 cm^{-1} as well as 1500 cm^{-1} and 1200cm^{-1}). Mostly a subtraction factor near one can be applied if samples contain a high protein content and if a placebo formulation is available at the same concentration and composition. However, if concentrations or compositions vary, the usage of more extreme values for the subtraction factor becomes necessary, thereby increasing the danger of artifacts within the spectrum. Subtraction can be considered successful if a flat baseline between 2000 cm^{-1} and 1800 cm^{-1} is accomplished and no excipient signal is visible anymore between 1500 cm^{-1} and 1200 cm^{-1}.

Any changes in protein secondary structure due to e.g. lyophilization stresses can be detected by comparing spectra of the untreated and the freeze-dried samples. A straight-forward procedure is calculation of the correlation coefficient "r" of the area normalized raw spectra or their 2nd derivatives (Fig. 3.4) [Arrondo et al. 1993; Kendrick et al. 1996]. The closer the calculated value is to 1, the better is the match of the two compared spectra.

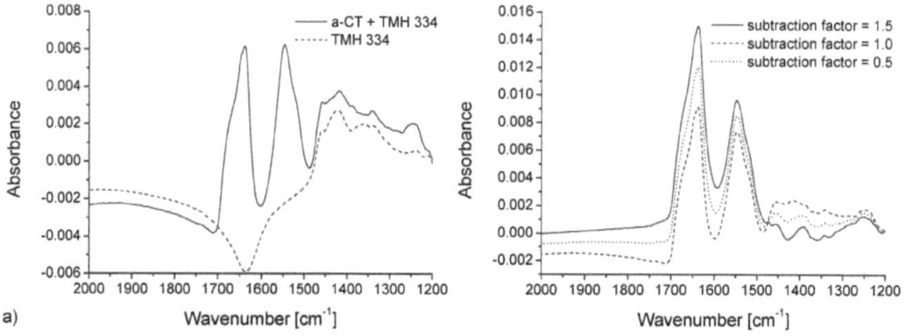

Fig. 3.3: a) Raw spectra of a mixture of protein and excipients and of excipients alone. b) Influence of subtraction factor on the shape of the final spectra [Vonhoff 2008].

Shifting and broadening of the amide I band due to lyophilization induced unfolding can easily and objectively be detected by this method [Pikal-Cleland et al. 2001]. However, detailed information about changes in protein secondary structure cannot be obtained. Also, a macroscopic comparison of the raw spectra is still necessary to identify false negative results due to baseline effects.

More information concerning structural changes can be obtained by subtracting the baseline corrected and area normalized amide I bands of the untreated and processed protein (Fig. 3.5). Any increase or decrease of the amide I band is visible within the difference spectrum. With knowledge in assigning wavenumbers to secondary structure elements, changes can easily be quantified by putting the integrated areas of the difference spectrum in relation to the area of the raw spectrum. However, information obtained remains rather vague because overlapping areas complicate differentiation between individual structural components.

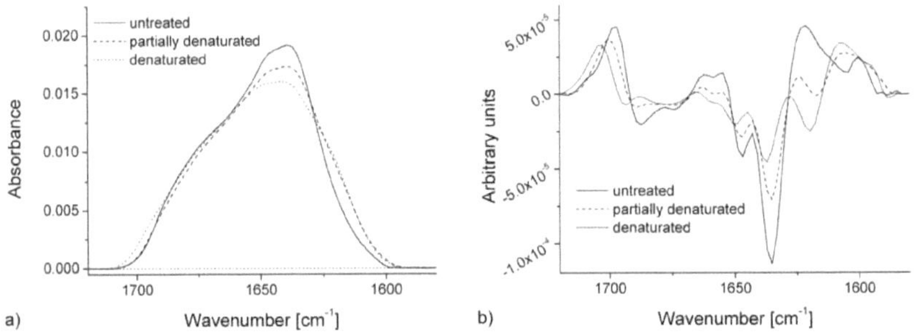

Fig. 3.4: a) Area normalized raw spectra of the amide I band of a-CT b) 2nd derivatives of the same spectra. During denaturation a decrease in overall intensity of individual structural features is visible in both spectra [Vonhoff 2009].

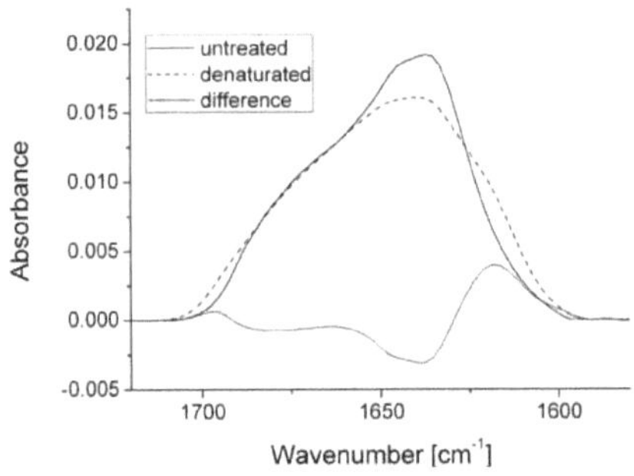

Fig. 3.5: Difference spectrum of native and heat treated a-CT. Integration of different parts of the difference spectrum can be used for quantifying spectral changes [Vonhoff 2009].

A further approach of detecting structural changes is peak fitting [Jackson et al. 1995]. Different secondary structure elements appear at defined wavenumbers, and their signal intensity correlates with their percentile content within the protein. As the amide I band consists of multiple superimposing peaks, its shape is rather poorly resolved. That's why the spectrum has to be preprocessed before quantification. Fourier Self-Deconvolution (FSD) and 2nd derivative spectra are often used to visualize overlapping peaks within the amide I region.

FSD is a band-narrowing technique that improves the outline of the band and thereby facilitates spectral interpretation (Fig. 3.6). The integrated areas of the component bands remain unaltered, and peak fitting can more easily be performed [Susi et al. 1985]. However, great care must be taken during FSD as the results are dependent on the factors chosen (bandwidth "w" and exponential "n") and a high amount of subjectivity is introduced.

2nd derivative spectra, on the other hand, offer an easy and objective way to qualitatively determine peak positions and numbers. Height and width of the individual peaks of the non-deconvolved spectrum, determined by either of the two aforementioned methods, can be calculated by an iteration process. The software tries to rebuild the amide I band based on the assumption that the sum of all peak areas gives the recorded spectrum (Fig. 3.7). Obviously, this technique is very time consuming and has some disadvantages:

- Due to the weak shape of the amide I band, more than just one peak fit is often possible.
- The fit is bound to be incorrect if not all peaks are placed correctly.
- Wrong assignment of peak positions and corresponding secondary structure elements will lead to false results.

The fourth approach for protein quantification using FTIR spectroscopy are pattern recognition techniques [Sarver et al. 1991; van der Weert et al. 2005]. The sample spectrum is compared with a set of standards with known secondary structures using principal component analysis, singular value decomposition or factor analysis. Failures due to false peak assignment are avoided and structural changes can be quantified objectively. On the downside, the information obtained is limited by the parameters included in the standards, and any errors during calibration will be present in the quantification procedure.

To be able to determine potential damage to protein secondary structure during spray-freeze-drying, a new pattern recognition technique that utilizes a partial least squares algorithm has been developed in this work (see chapter 4.5). During its calibration, native as well as denaturated conformations were included. This way, the aforementioned problems during the quantification of protein secondary structure could be avoided, while still delivering a high level of information regarding protein denaturation and aggregation.

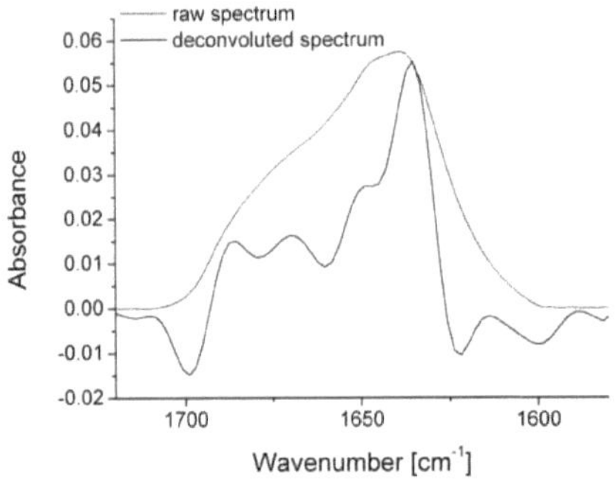

Fig. 3.6: Raw and FSD spectra of α-chymotrypsin (n = 2,4; width = 30) [Vonhoff 2009].

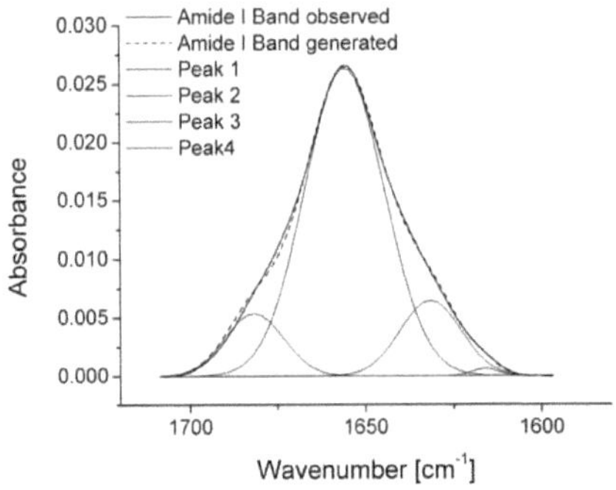

Fig. 3.7: Peak fit of human serum albumin in aqueous solution at pH 7.0. Second derivative spectra only revealed 4 peaks within the amide I band [Vonhoff 2009].

4. Materials and methods

4.1 Model Proteins

α-Chymotrypsin (a-CT) and human serum albumin (HSA) were used as model proteins during the SFD experiments performed in this work and therefore will receive a detailed biological description in this chapter. Other proteins used as standards during the generation of the FTIR calibration curve are listed in chapter 4.2.

α-Chymotrypsin

a-CT belongs to the family of serin proteases which cleave the amide function within a polypeptide into two new smaller peptides. To facilitate this reaction, the active center of the enzyme consists of a catalytic triad formed by the three side chains asparagine, histidine and serin. In this constellation, histidine can stabilize serin during its nucleophile reaction with the peptide bond of the substrate. Asparagine further enhances the proton uptake ability of histidine. The resulting instable tetrahedron intermediate is stabilized within the "oxanion hole". From there on, the amide bond is cleaved, and one part of the peptide is attached to the enzyme while the other diffuses. Finally, the enzyme-peptide intermediate is being hydrolyzed and thus the catalyst is restored. Selectivity for the position of the amide bond of the substrate is rather low with a slight preference for the amino acids tryptophane, tyrosine and phenylalanine [Stryer et al. 2008].

Chymotrypsinogen is the inactive precursor protein of α-chymotrypsin and comprises 245 amino acids. During its activation the residues 14 – 15 and 147 – 148 are excised which leaves behind three peptide chains held together by various disulfide bonds. Those chains are arranged into two domains, each containing about 120 amino acids folded mostly as antiparallel β-sheets (Fig. 4.1a).

α-Chymotrypsin exhibits a molecular weight of approximately 25 kDa and has an optimal pH value of 7.8 with an isoelectric point (IEP) of 8.75. Increasing or decreasing the pH from its optimum to 9.3 or 6.0 leads to a drop in enzyme activity to 35% and 40%, respectively.

a-CT is both activated and stabilized by Ca^{2+} and is still active in the presence of denaturants like 0.1% SDS (sodiumdodecylsulfat) and 2M guanidine hydrochloride. However, the activity of a-CT can be inhibited by the addition of several substances like chymostatin, aprotinin, α_1-antitrypsin and α_2-macroglobulin. Its temperature optimum lies at 50°C [Sigma-Aldrich 2009].

Human serum albumin

Human serum albumin is the most abundant protein in human serum and exhibits a highly helical secondary structure. It is divided into three homologous helical domains (I, II and III) which are stabilized by an internal network of disulfide bonds. Each domain has two subdomains with a common helical motif (Fig. 4.1b). The structural domains are covalently connected by peptide bonds into a single polypeptide chain with 585 amino acid residues [Wang et al. 2005]. The protein is synthesized in the liver as prepro-albumin and then transformed into mature albumin by the removal of several amino acids from its N-terminus.

HSA exhibits a molecular mass of 69 kDa and serves multiple purposes inside the human body. For one, HSA plays a major part in providing the osmotic pressure in plasma simply due to its high concentration [Walsh 2001]. Additionally, HSA serves as multifunctional transport protein for many small organic and inorganic molecules. Ibuprofen and phenylbutazone, for example, can reversibly bind to specific regions within the protein (binding sites I and II). Binding sites for other molecules, such as fatty acids, bilirubin or metal ions, exist as well [Roswell 2008].

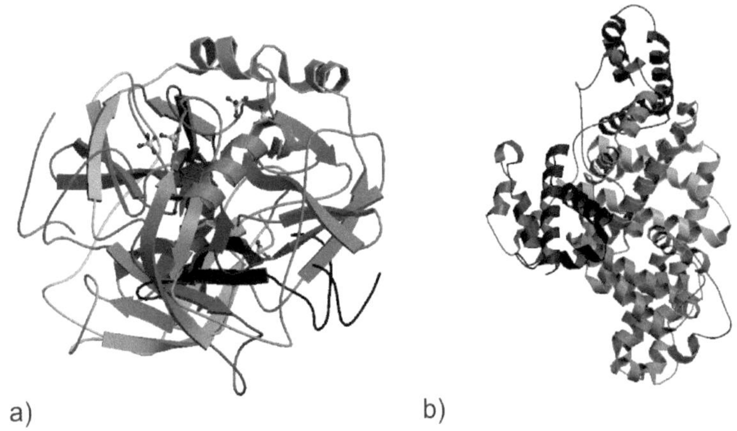

Fig. 4.1: 3D structures of a) α-chymotrypsin and b) human serum albumin. Pictures taken from RCSB Protein Data Bank [Berman et al. 2000]

Apart from its physiological application, HSA has also previously been used to stabilize other proteins during freeze-drying. It can sustain comparably high temperatures (up to 10 h at 60°C), shows good solubility and undergoes many reversible conformational changes during pH shifts [Wang 1988]. Below a pH of 3, the protein is converted into the "E" form (expanded). With increasing pH, HSA first transforms into the "F" form (for moving "fast" during gel electrophoresis at pH 3 – 4) and then into the "N" form (normal) at pH 4.3. Finally, by increasing the pH even further, HSA is transformed into the "B" (basic) form. Those transitions are mainly caused by the rupture of intramolecular ionic pairs due to the pH shifts [Barone 1992].

4.2 Excipients and reagents

All proteins used for creating the iPLS algorithm for FTIR spectroscopy are summarized in Table 4.1. Any reagents and solvents used for the spray-freeze-drying experiments as well as other substances needed for analysis of the resulting SFD products are presented in Table 4.2.

Table 4.1: Proteins used as standards for creating the FTIR calibration curves.

Proteins	Lot-No.	Supplied by
Alkaline phosphatase from bovine intestinal mucosa	075K7012	Sigma, Germany (P7640)
Bovine serum albumin	038K0665	Sigma, Germany (A7906)
Carbonic anhydrase from bovine erythrocytes	078K1181	Sigma, Germany (C3934)
Carboxypeptidase A from bovine pancreas	105K7770	Sigma, Germany (C9268)
Catalase from bovine liver	046K7046	Sigma, Germany (C1345)
Concanavalin A from Canavalia ensiformis	066K7031	Sigma, Germany (C2010)
α-Chymotrypsin from bovine pancreas	086K7695 105K7670	Sigma, Germany (C4129)
β-Galactosidase from bovine liver	045H7025	Sigma, Germany (G1875)
Glucagon	065K1027	Sigma, Germany (G2044)
Hemoglobin from bovine blood	010K7618	Sigma, Germany (H2500)
Human serum albumin	095K7588	Sigma, Germany (A9511)
Insulin from bovine pancreas	096K1527	Sigma, Germany (I5500)
L-Lactic dehydrogenase from rabbit muscle	1245674 14907241	Fluka, Switzerland (61309)
Lysozyme from chicken egg white	91K7021	Sigma, Germany (L7651)
Myoglobin from equine skeletal muscle	028K7002	Sigma, Germany (M0630)
Ribonuclease A from bovine pancreas	128K7002	Sigma, Germany (R6513)

Table 4.2: Reagents and solvents used in this thesis.

Reagent / solvent	Lot-No.	Supplied by
Ammonium iron(II) sulfate hexahydrate	03128AJ-108	Sigma, Germany (215406)
N-Benzoyl-L-tyrosine ethyl ester	085K1656	Sigma, Germany (B6125)
Calcium chloride dihydrate	31K251	Sigma, Germany (C3881)
(1*R*)-(-)-10-Camphorsulfonic acid ammonium salt	11606TD-239	Sigma, Germany(21369)
Dextran from Leuconostoc mesenteroides	1331472 41107018	Sigma, Germany (D9260)
Hydrochloric acid	K37709617 732	Merck, Germany (1003171000)
Hydroxyethyl starch Pentastarch	02432	Fresenius Kabi, Germany
Mannitol	E888Y	Roquette, France
Methanol	627911	Roth, Germany (7342.1)
Potassium Iodide	81860	Sigma, Germany (30315)
Sucrose	096K0026	Sigma, Germany (S9378)
Terephthalic acid	01705TH-278	Sigma, Germany (185361)
D-(+)-Trehalose dihydrate	114K7064	Sigma, Germany (T9449)
Trisma® base	018K5423	Sigma, Germany (T1503)

4.3 Spray-freezing into vapor over liquid

4.3.1 Experimental setup

The experimental setup previously described by Gieseler et al. [2009] was modified in order to manufacture SFD particles from multiple formulations and atomization conditions during one freeze-drying cycle, thus making the process less time-consuming. In short, the liquid feed (1) was forwarded by a peristaltic pump bearing 10 rollers (2) to an ultrasound nozzle (3). From there it was atomized into an insulated bowl (4) (Fig. 4.2a) containing LN_2 (Fig. 4.2b). After the spraying step, the gauge was opened and the suspended frozen droplets could be transferred into 20 mL freeze-drying vials (5).

In contrast to the work by Gieseler et al. [2009], the volume of the bowl was drastically reduced which made filling of the resulting suspension quantitatively into a single vial possible. After rinsing once with LN_2 it could be reused for a different preparation thus improving feasibility of the experimental setup. Even more important, the fill volume of the vial could be adjusted precisely as it was only determined by the volume of the atomized formulation.

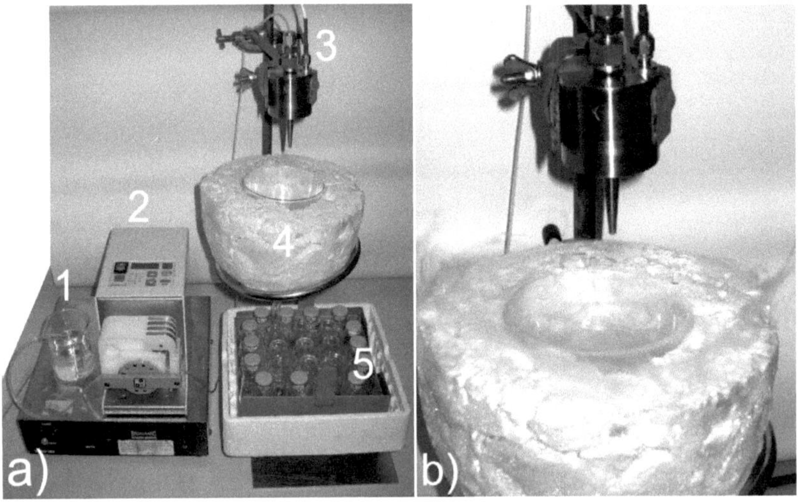

Fig. 4.2: Experimental setup for producing SFD particles. a) Complete setup b) Close-up view during spraying into liquid nitrogen.

This resulted in improved reproducibility of primary and secondary drying times during lyophilization. The custom-made mini-tray visible in Fig. 4.2a presents the second important improvement over the earlier SFD setup yielding multiple advantages:

1. Just like in classic freeze-drying experiments, the outer vials serve as radiation shield during lyophilization. This decreases the edge vial effect thus improving reproducibility of the drying step [Rambhatla et al. 2003].
2. By using all of the inner vials, up to nine different formulations or process conditions can be lyophilized per run.
3. Loading times of the freeze-dryer are substantially reduced in comparison to inserting the vials separately, thus leading to reduced water vapor condensation and ice formation on the shelves of the freeze-dryer.
4. Vials are kept in place with help of the tray while the last remains of cryogen are boiled off. Otherwise the vials tend to move around the shelves during this step, possibly tilting over.

As the spraying step could take more than one hour, depending on the number of individual preparations, the tray was kept inside a polystyrene box filled with cryogen to prevent the frozen droplets from melting (Fig. 4.2a). Subsequent to the atomization period, LN_2 was boiled off (see chapter 4.3.2) and the tray was transferred into the freeze-dryer.

4.3.2 Freeze-drying

Lyophilization was performed on a Virtis Advantage Plus benchtop scale freeze-dryer (Fig. 4.3). Vials were quickly transferred from the experimental SFD setup onto the pre-cooled shelves (-50°C) of the freeze-dryer with help of the mini-tray described above.

Four FDPS type "T" (Cu / constantan) thermocouples (SP Industries, Warminster, USA) were used for monitoring product temperatures and thus determining the endpoint of primary and secondary drying. Slight variations were observed, regarding the fill volume of the vials. This was caused by inhomogeneity during the atomization step where a part of the droplet fraction was lost after freezing on the bowl surface. Therefore, a "failsafe" freeze-drying cycle was designed which was characterized by prolonged drying times in combination with a very slow ramping step into secondary drying.

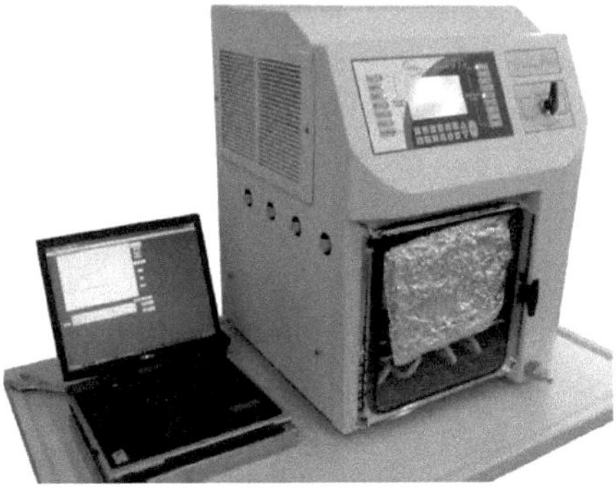

Fig. 4.3: Virtis Advantage Plus freeze-dryer.

Fig. 4.4 presents a representative FD run recorded during a SFD experiment using three different high concentrated a-CT formulations and one placebo preparation. As soon as temperatures inside the vials started to rise, last remnants of LN_2 were considered removed, and ramping to the primary drying settings was initiated (to -24°C, 70 mTorr within 20 min). This was especially important as the Virtis freeze-dryer automatically applied a slight vacuum to seal its door when the program was started.

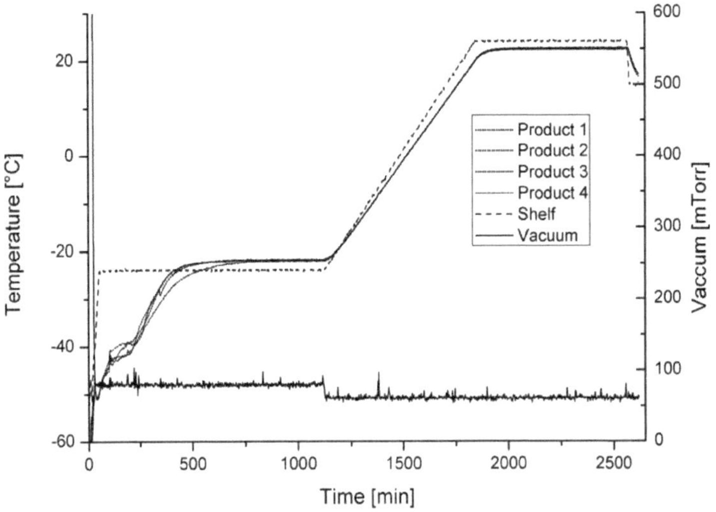

Fig. 4.4: Standard freeze-drying cycle used throughout all SFD experiments.

This would lead to strong boiling retardation if LN_2 was still present inside the vials. Conditions during primary drying were then held constant for up to 36 h. To reduce cycle times, ramping into secondary drying (to +24°C, 0.07°C/min) was triggered manually if all product temperature recordings had already exceeded shelf temperatures at an earlier point.

Secondary drying was performed for additional 12 h at +24°C and 50 mTorr. After the cycle was finished, the freeze-dryer was flushed with nitrogen and the vials were immediately transferred into glove boxes with a relative humidity (rh) of < 1% at a temperature of 20°C. Throughout the cycle the condenser temperature was constantly maintained below -65°C. An aluminum foil was inserted between shelf and the door of the freeze-dryer to shield the product from elevated heat radiation [Schneid et al. 2008].

4.3.3 Nozzles

The nozzles investigated in this thesis mostly achieve atomization by the means of ultrasound. Fig. 4.5a-d shows four different types of ultrasonic nozzles operating at frequencies of 25 kHz, 48 kHz, 60 kHz and 120 kHz respectively. Disc-shaped ceramic piezoelectric transducers convert high-frequency electrical energy into vibratory mechanical motion at the same frequency (Fig. 4.5e). The excitation created by the transducers produces transversal standing waves along the longitudinal axis of the nozzle which are absorbed by the liquid. At a critical amplitude cohesion of the fluid is overcome and atomization finally occurs. The vibration amplitude is greatest at the antinode of the standing wave. Using nozzle lengths that are a multiple of a half-wavelength, this effect can be exploited which simplifies atomization [Sono-Tek 2005].

Being designed for operation inside a standard spray-dryer, the 25 kHz nozzle is surrounded by an outer hull, revealing only the very end of the nozzle tip. As one can see, the front horn becomes consecutively shorter with increasing atomization frequency. This is caused by the fact that wavelengths become shorter with increasing nozzle frequencies. Therefore, the nozzle length must be reduced if vibration at the antinode shall still be used.

The right level of power input is essential for successful spraying. Below a certain power, there is insufficient energy available for atomization, while at too high power inputs cavitation occurs, literally ripping the solution apart. Atomization is usually performed at power inputs between 1 Watts and 15 Watts with higher viscosities and liquid feed rates generally requiring higher power values [Sono-Tek 2005]. Droplet size is governed by the nozzle frequency with higher frequencies resulting in smaller droplets.

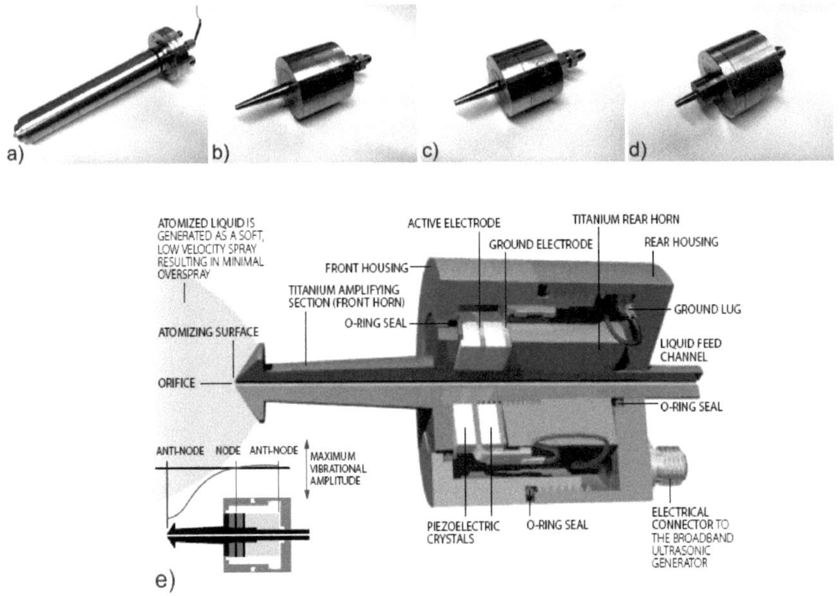

Fig. 4.5: Ultrasonic nozzles used in this work, operating at different frequencies. a) 25 kHz nozzle, b) 48 kHz nozzle, c) 60 kHz nozzle, d) 120 kHz nozzle, e) schematics of an ultrasound nozzle [Sono-Tek 2009].

For example, Schiffter [2007] was able to produce SFD particles with a $d_{v,0.5}$ of 53.12 µm and a very narrow span of 0.646 by spraying a high concentrated trehalose/mannitol/dextran solution with a 25 kHz nozzle. By applying a 48 kHz nozzle instead, the $d_{v,0.5}$ decreased to 46.81 µm while span increased to 0.921. The biggest advantage of ultrasound nozzles over its two-fluid counterpart is that they produce a so-called "soft spray". This means that droplets travel at low velocities without a propelling air flow. As a result, the feasibility of the SFD experiment is improved, because the agitation of LN_2 during spraying is strongly reduced [Sonner 2002]. Ultrasound nozzles are available in different modifications for influencing the shape of the spray as well as options for heating/cooling of the nozzle core, adding thermocouples, etc. However, these variations are not covered in this chapter as SFD experiments were performed using ultrasound nozzles in their basic setup.

The second type of nozzle used in this thesis was a two-fluid nozzle designed for operation inside a laboratory spray-dryer. Atomization is performed by a pressurized gas-flow that rips the solution apart, thereby creating the fine droplet spray. Droplet sizes can be controlled by adjusting liquid feed rate and atomizing air flow [Masters 1991].

4.4 Nozzle characterization

4.4.1 Temperature measurements

In contrast to two-fluid nozzles, ultrasonic nozzles generate a spray of fine droplets by oscillation of a piezoelectric crystal. Part of the energy input is inevitably transformed into heat dissipation which leads to increasing temperatures during the atomization step. As proteins are often heat-sensitive, evaluation of the temperature is an important factor for the characterization of ultrasound nozzles [Scharnagl et al. 2005]. However, determination of the heat output is problematic as measurements directly inside the nozzle suffer from severe noise, while temperatures on the outside of the nozzle body were generally considered too low. Therefore, a thermocouple was placed directly underneath the nozzle orifice measuring the spray temperatures (Fig. 4.6).

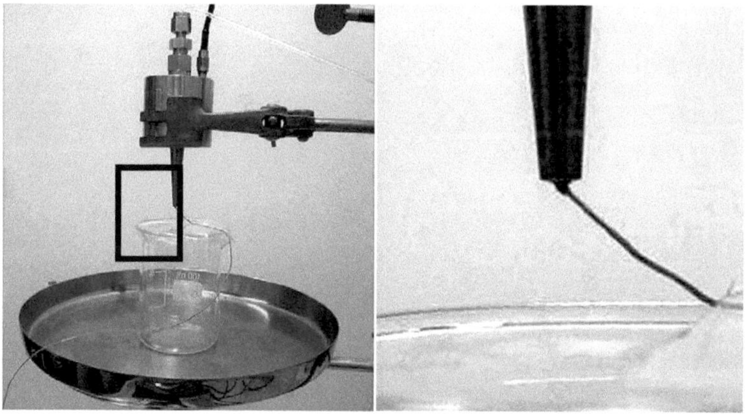

Fig. 4.6: Experimental setup for recording the temperature-time-profile of four different ultrasonic nozzles. The thermocouple was placed directly beneath the nozzle orifice.

Laboratory air conditioning kept the ambient temperature at 22°C throughout all experiments. The heat output of four different ultrasonic nozzles (25 kHz, 48 kHz, 60 kHz, 120 kHz) was evaluated by generating a temperature-time-profile. Temperature measurements were performed equal to SFD experiments using a peristaltic pump with 6 rollers. Double distilled and filtered water (0.2 µm) was pumped at a liquid feed rate of 1 mL/min. Data was recorded at a 5 seconds time interval using an Omega OM-CP-QuadTEMP data logger (Omega Engineering Inc., CT, USA). After 12 minutes steady-state temperatures had been achieved for all investigated nozzles, and data recording was stopped.

4.4.2 Cavitation experiments

The occurrence of cavitation was investigated for the 25 kHz, 48 kHz, 60 kHz and 120 kHz nozzles. During cavitation, ultrasound agitation generates small air bubbles within a fluid that experience a quasi-adiabatic collapse after reaching a certain size. This leads to locally high temperatures and pressures as well as irradiation of acoustic shockwaves [Sponer 1990]. Under these conditions, free radicals are formed that can react with the protein solutions during atomization [van de Weert et al. 2000] and thus lead to chemical instabilities (see chapter 2.2.2). For analytical purposes, the in-situ generated free radicals can be used to oxidize marker solutions. Potassium iodide (KI), terephthalic acid (TA) or Fricke reagent (Fe*)* have been used in the past to quantify the extent of cavitation by oxidation (see Equation 4.1 to Equation 4.3) [McLean et al. 1988; Koda et al. 2003].

Equation 4.1 $I^{-} + OH\cdot \rightarrow I\cdot + OH^{-}$ and $2I\cdot \rightarrow I_2$

Equation 4.2 $Fe^{2+} + OH\cdot \rightarrow Fe^{3+} + OH^{-}$

Equation 4.3 $TA + OH\cdot \rightarrow HTA + OH^{-}$

where HTA stands for hydroxyterephthalic acid.

For KI and Fe, increases in absorbances were determined at 355 nm and 304 nm respectively using the PerkinElmer Lambda 25 spectrometer described in chapter 4.6.1. Fluorescence emission intensity of HTA at 425 nm was determined with an excitation wavelength of 315 nm using the PerkinElmer LS 55 fluorimeter described in chapter 4.6.2.

Potassium iodide was dissolved in double distilled and filtered water (0.2 µm) at a concentration of 0.2 mmol/l. The 4 mmol/l terephthalic acid solution was prepared by dissolving the reagent in double distilled and filtered water (0.2 µm) and adding enough 1 M NaOH to adjust the pH to 7.3. Finally, Fricke reagent solution was prepared by diluting 96% (w/w) H_2SO_4 to 0.4 mol/l and then dissolving 4 mmol NaCl and 4 mmol ammonium iron(II) sulfate hexahydrate in one litre of the diluted sulfuric acid.

As stated in chapter 4.3.3, atomization was performed at the tip of the nozzle where the anti-node of the transverse standing wave is located. It seems obvious that cavitation must occur in this region rather than inside the nozzle body. For that reason, only the nozzle orifice was immersed into the test solutions (see Fig. 4.7). As a result, no loss in the fine droplet fraction could be observed during the experiments which improved quantitative evaluations. On the other hand, these changes constituted a difference to the usual SFD setup where atomization was performed a few centimeters above the cryogen. Nevertheless, this setup proved feasible to compare cavitation stress during the spraying step.

20 mL of the marker solution were filled into a Petri dish. The nozzle was immersed into the liquid and slightly lifted up again until its tip was positioned barely below the surface to ensure flawless functioning. The nozzle was operated for four minutes. Each experiment was performed in triplicate and evaluated by average and standard deviation values.

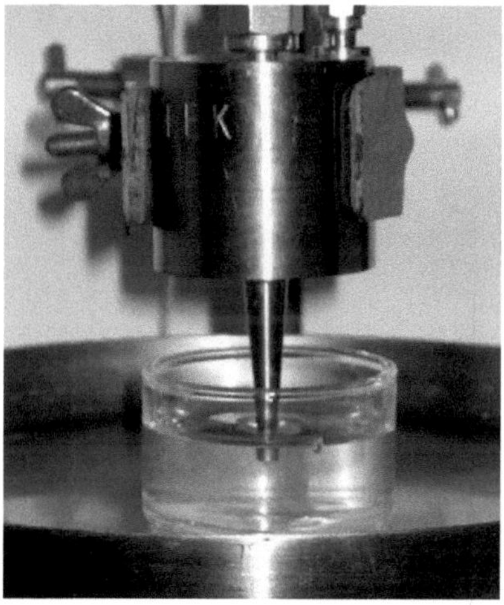

Fig. 4.7: Experimental setup for determining cavitation effects by different ultrasound nozzles.

4.5 FTIR

4.5.1 Mathematical Background

The mathematical methods used for correlating the measured absorbance of a sample with the concentrations of its individual constituents have been extensively discussed in literature [Dousseau et al. 1990; Kalnin et al. 1990; Lee et al. 1990]. The most important approaches used in thesis are shortly described in the following sections.

4.5.1.1 Classic least squares (CLS)

The simplest approach is directly based in Beer's Law: The measured absorbance at a given wavelength A_λ is directly proportional to its extinction coefficient ε_λ, the pathlength of light b and the constituent concentration c (Equation 4.4).

Equation 4.4 $$A_\lambda = \varepsilon_\lambda \cdot c \cdot b$$

If the measurements are performed at a fixed wavelength Equation 4.4 can further be simplified to Equation 4.5:

Equation 4.5 $$A_\lambda = K_\lambda \cdot c$$

During calibration the equation is solved for K_λ and unknown concentrations can be calculated from their absorbencies. By measuring samples at a series of different concentrations followed by least squares regression, errors due to noise or sample handling can be overcome. If more than one constituent is present, multiple calibration curves have to be generated. However, if strongly overlapping components must be quantified (like the different secondary structure peaks within the amide I band) this classic approach has to be further modified. As Beer's Law is additive, the equations for a single spectrum at two different wavelengths would be

Equation 4.6 $$A_{\lambda 1} = K_{a,\lambda 1} \cdot C_a + K_{b\lambda 1} \cdot C_b$$

and

Equation 4.7 $$A_{\lambda 2} = K_{a,\lambda 2} \cdot C_a + K_{b\lambda 2} \cdot C_b$$

After introducing two more variables for errors during measurements ($E_{\lambda 1}$ and $E_{\lambda 2}$) the equations can also be rewritten as matrix:

Equation 4.8 $$\begin{vmatrix} A_{\lambda 1} \\ A_{\lambda 2} \end{vmatrix} = \begin{vmatrix} K_{a,\lambda 1} & K_{b,\lambda 1} \\ K_{a,\lambda 2} & K_{b,\lambda 2} \end{vmatrix} \begin{vmatrix} C_a \\ C_b \end{vmatrix} + \begin{vmatrix} E_{\lambda 1} \\ E_{\lambda 2} \end{vmatrix}$$

or in short

Equation 4.9 $$A = K \cdot C + E$$

Equation 4.9 can be used for calibration by solving for K:

Equation 4.10 $$K = AC^T(CC^T)^{-1}$$

where T indicates the transpose of a matrix, and $C^T(CC^T)^{-1}$ is the so-called pseudo-inverse.

CLS is a fast and straightforward approach. However, as absorbance is calculated as the sum of absorbance of the individual components, the concentration of each constituent (even nonsignificant ones) has to be known during calibration. Baseline effects and interactions between the components also lead to false quantifications. Due to these reasons CLS is usually not applied for quantifying protein secondary structure.

4.5.1.2 *Inverse least squares (ILS)*

ILS does not require knowledge of every constituent inside the sample to calculate the correct matrix of coefficients K and is therefore different from CLS.

A and C can be related, in matrix form, using

Equation 4.11 $$A^T K = C^T$$

This way the concentration is expressed as a function of the absorbance at a series of different wavelengths. This is completely different to CLS where absorbance at a single wavelength is calculated as an additive function of the constituent concentrations. A solution which minimizes the squared error may be sought by differentiating Equation 4.11, which, after a little manipulation, yields a solution for K which takes the form of

Equation 4.12 $$K = (AA^T)^{-1} AC^T$$

This allows us to evaluate K, which may be used to calculate the concentrations of new spectra, $\underline{c}$, from a measured set of absorbencies, $\underline{a}$, such that

Equation 4.13 $$\underline{c} = K^T \underline{a}$$

Unfortunately, the quantity $(AA^T)^{-1}A$ from Equation 4.12 is computationally inefficient to calculate. A number of algorithms exist to accurately approximate the values of $(AA^T)^{-1}A$ and these have been used extensively to calculate structure concentrations in the past [Rahmelow et al. 1996; Forato et al. 1998; Wang et al. 2008]. Two algorithms of interest are presented here in summary. The reader may wish to refer to the theoretical comparison of these two methods by Lorber for a more detailed description [Lorber 1987].

Singular value decomposition (SVD):

SVD is a combination of inverse least-squares and principal component analysis. Unlike quantification methods that are based directly on Beer's Law, SVD regresses the structural contents from variance spectra U ("eigenvectors") and its loading factors ("scores"). This means that with SVD the absorbance matrix is decomposed during a first step into its eigenvectors and scores. These are used in a second step to calculate the absorptivity constants by an inverse least-squares algorithm. This way the efficiency of matrix calculations is improved as unnecessary information is being removed.

First, A is decomposed into three matrices and rewritten as

Equation 4.14 $$A = USV^T$$

Where U and V are orthogonal and S is diagonal, containing the singular values s_{ii}. Calculations are simplified further by removing vectors corresponding to small singular values from U,S and V, reducing their rank and leading to

Equation 4.15 $$A \approx U_1 S_1 V_1^T$$

This approximation to A can be substituted into Equation 4.12, providing a new estimate for K which can be written as

Equation 4.16 $$K^T = U_1 S_1^{-1} V_1^T C^T$$

Partial least squares (PLS)

PLS is a quantitative decomposition technique that is closely related to SVD, but is often more robust, especially when a high degree of multicollinearity exists between elements of the C matrix. The main difference between both algorithms is that PLS decomposes both the spectral data and the structural contents, giving two sets of vectors and scores: The matrices A and C are redefined as $A=TP^T$ and $C^T=UQ^T$. As the spectral information and the secondary structures are connected, the two sets of scores can be related to each other by regression ($U=TV$) and a calibration model can be constructed [Vonhoff et al. 2009]. Spectral decomposition and regression are performed in one step. The precision of evaluation can be further enhanced by defining limits for critical regions of individual secondary structures ("intervals") thus reducing the influence of regions containing noise or high levels of collinearitiy. The interval partial least squares algorithm is employed for determining protein secondary structure throughout this thesis.

4.5.2 Sample recording

Protein spectra were recorded on an Omnic Nicolet MagnaIR 550 spectrometer (Thermo Fisher Scientific Inc., Germany) (Fig. 4.8a) equipped with a DTGS KBr detector and a KBr beamsplitter at a resolution of 4 cm^{-1}. The apparatus was constantly purged with dry air (1 bar) to eliminate any artifacts by water vapor. All samples were collected using a Proteus CaF_2 transmission cell (Thermo Fisher Scientific Inc., Germany) with an optical path length of 6 µm (Fig. 4.8b). In the advanced options tab of the Omnic 7.2 recording software, zero filling was set to "0" while "Happ-Genzel" and "Mertz" were chosen for apodization and phase correction, respectively. For each measurement a total of 42 scans was collected at slowest mirror speeds possible to minimize spectral noise. The measurements were repeated three times and averaged to reduce baseline effects. Between measurements the cell was first purged with 1M hydrochloric acid followed by pure water until no signal of the sample was detectable anymore. The sample could be injected into the transmission cell without having to open the measurement chamber by connecting it via two Luer lock tubings. This drastically reduced measurement times as the chamber did not have to be conditioned again to the same rh values. Subtraction of the background signal was performed manually with a subtraction factor usually between 0.95 and 1.05 until a flat baseline between 1900 cm^{-1} and 1740 cm^{-1} was reached [Chittur 1998]. Placebo formulations for background subtraction were prepared simultaneously with the protein samples in the same SFD run. To improve the quality of the subtraction spectrum, both protein and placebo formulation were recorded at the same concentrations. The spectral region between 1500 cm^{-1} and 1100 cm^{-1} was used to evaluate the quality of the subtraction spectra. The protein spectrum of a formulation was considered free of excipients if no artifacts were visible compared to the pure samples.

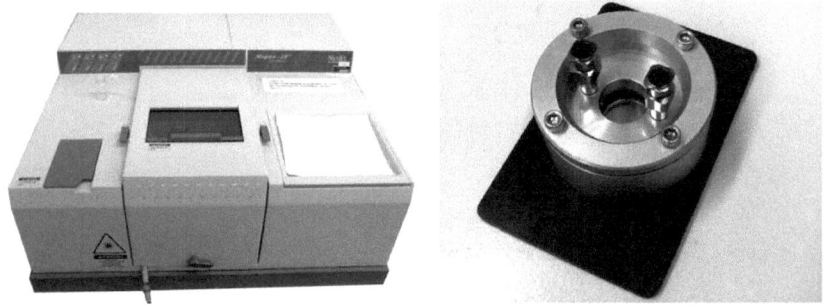

Fig. 4.8: a) Omnic Magna IR550 spectrometer b) Proteus cell transmission kit.

4.6 Additional analytical methods

4.6.1 UV/VIS spectroscopy activity assay

α-Chymotrypsin enzyme activity was evaluated on a PerkinElmer Lambda 25 UV/Vis spectrometer by continuous spectrophotometric rate determination according to Wirnt [1974]. In this assay, chymotrypsin catalyzes the hydrolysis of N-benzoyl-L-tyrosin ethyl ester (BTEE) into N-benzoyl-L-tyrosin (BT) and ethanol (Equation 4.17). One unit hydrolyzes 1.0 μmol of BTEE per minute at pH 7.8 at 25°C and the increase of BT is measured by observing the increase in absorbance at 256 nm.

Equation 4.17 $$BTEE + H_2O \xrightarrow{chymotrypsin} BT + ethanol$$

The spectrometer was connected to a PC with PerkinElmer UV WinLab 5.0 software (PerkinElmer LAS GmbH; Rodgau, Germany) and changes in absorbance were recorded for three minutes while a waterbath was used to keep the quartz cuvette (3 mL, b=1 cm) at 25°C. Before measurements, a 80mM Tris Buffer was prepared and adjusted to pH 7.8 at 25°C with 1M HCl. The BTEE solution was manufactured by initially dissolving 1.18 mM of the substrate in 31.7 mL MeOH and then adding water until the final volume was 50 mL. Finally, a 2M $CaCl_2$ solution was prepared that served as stabilizer during the assay. Immediately before each measurement 1.42 mL buffer, 1.40 mL substrate and 0.08 mL $CaCl_2$ solution were mixed by inversion inside the cuvette and then equilibrated to 25°C. Afterwards, 0.1 mL of an a-CT solution were added containing 2-5 units/mL of enzyme (assuming an undamaged protein) and once again mixed by inversion. The final 3 mL reaction mixture consisted of 38 mM Tris, 0.55 mM N-benzoyl-L-tyrosine ethyl ester, 30% (v/v) methanol, 53 mM calcium chloride, 0.03 mM hydrochloric acid and 0.2 - 0.5 units of chymotrypsin.

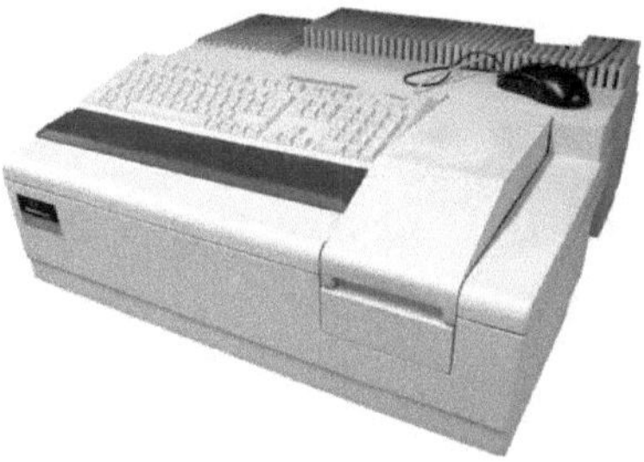

Fig. 4.9: PerkinElmer Lambda 25 UV/Vis spectrometer.

For each batch of samples a new untreated standard was quantified and set to 100% to compensate for fluctuations in the composition of the reagent mixture. From the increase in absorbance during one minute ($\Delta A_{256nm/60sec}$), the residual enzyme activity can be calculated by Equation 4.18.

Equation 4.18 $$Units\,/\,ml_{enzyme} = \frac{\Delta A_{256nm/60\sec} \cdot 3 \cdot df}{0.964 \cdot 0.1}$$

where 3 is the final volume of the assay in mL, df is the dilution factor, 0.964 is the millimolar extinction coefficient of N-benzoyl-L-tyrosine at 256 nm, and 0.1 is the volume of enzyme used in mL.

The result can be used to calculate the $units_{enzyme}/mg_{solid}$ by Equation 4.19

Equation 4.19 $$units_{enzyme}\,/\,mg_{solid} = \frac{units_{enzyme}\,/\,ml_{enzyme}}{mg_{solid}\,/\,ml_{enzyme}}$$

while $units_{enzyme}/mg_{protein}$ can be determined by Equation 4.20.

Equation 4.20
$$units_{enzyme} / mg_{protein} = \frac{units_{enzyme} / ml_{enyzme}}{mg_{protein} / ml_{enzyme}}$$

All measurements were performed in triplicate and mean and sdv values were calculated.

4.6.2 Fluorescence spectroscopy

Protein tertiary structure was analyzed by intrinsic tryptophan fluorescence. Tryptophan has been the most popular marker in the past as its indole chromophore is highly sensitive to the polarity of its environment and shows a comparably high fluorescence quantum yield [Chen et al. 1998]. Apart from the tryptophan residue, tryrosine and phenylalanine are known to exhibit fluorescence as well within proteins. The wavelength of the fluorescence emission maximum (λ_{max}) ranges from 308 nm (like in azurin) to 355 nm (e.g. in glucagon) and roughly correlates with the degree of solvent exposure of the chromophore [Vivian et al. 2001]. The difference between excitation and fluorescence wavelength is called Stokes shift and is caused by solvent effects. A fluorophore undergoes changes in its polarity upon excitation towards a larger dipole moment. Following excitation the solvent molecules can re-orient around the fluorophore which lowers the energy of the excited state [Lakowicz 2006]. An approximation for describing the extent of the Stokes shift is given by Lippert-Mataga equation (Equation 4.21).

Equation 4.21
$$\bar{\nu}_A - \bar{\nu}_F = \frac{2}{hc}\left(\frac{\varepsilon - 1}{2\varepsilon + 1} - \frac{n^2 - 1}{2n^2 + 1}\right)\frac{(\mu_E - \mu_G)}{a^3} + const$$

where $\bar{\nu}_a$ and $\bar{\nu}_F$ are the wavenumbers [cm^{-1}] of absorption and emission, h is Planck's constant, c is the speed of light, ε is the dielectric constant and n the refractive index of the solvent, μ_E and μ_G are the dipole in the excited and ground state and a is the radius of the cavity in which the fluorophore resides. The term in the large parentheses is referred to as orientation polarizability (Δf). The first part of the term (ε-1) / (2ε+1) accounts for spectral shifts due to the reorientation of solvent dipoles and to redistribution of the electrons in the solvent phase while the second part (n^2 -1) / ($2n^2$+1) accounts only for the redistribution of electrons [Lakowicz 2006]. The redistribution of electrons happens so quickly that it effects both absorption and emission energies and therefore must be subtracted from the first term. It becomes apparent that orientation polarization increases during protein denaturation as the environment of tryptophan becomes more hydrophilic. Although the Lippert-Mataga equation is only an approximation, it readily describes the mechanism of increasing Stokes shifts during protein denaturation.

In summary, this means that a fluorophore exhibiting a noticeable change in dipole moment (μ_E-μ_G), like tryptophan, will show increasing bathochrome shifts if it is moved towards more hydrophilic environments. This is the case during denaturation, where the folding pattern of a protein is lost and tryptophan residues, originally buried at the inside of the protein, are located towards the outside.

The PerkinElmer LS55 fluorimeter (Fig. 4.10) was connected to a PC via FLWINLAB 4.0 software (PerkinElmer LAS GmbH; Rodgau, Germany). As fluorescence is temperature sensitive, the sample chamber was connected with a water bath set to 25°C throughout all experiments. Sample fluorescence was recorded from a low volume quartz cuvette at an angle of 90° and a scan speed of 150 nm/sec after temperature equilibration. The excitation wavelength was set to 295 nm by a monochromator, using a slit width of 10 nm. This way any bias by the excitation of tyrosine and phenylalanine was greatly reduced while keeping a good signal-to-noise ratio. The emission monochromator was used at varying slit widths depending on the intensity of the fluorescence signal. No polarization was applied by any of the monochromators. Every measurement was performed in triplicate and spectra were averaged to improve the signal-to-noise ratio. For comparison reasons, the average spectra were then normalized so that the maximum between 330 and 360 nm equaled 100 arbitrary units. Finally, the positions of the spectral maxima were determined automatically by FLWINLAB.

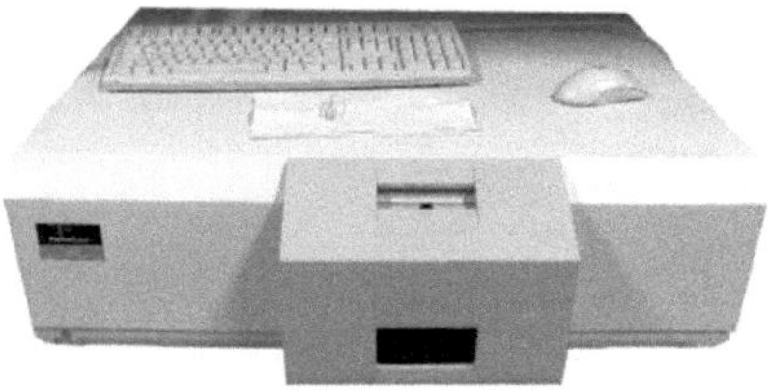

Fig. 4.10: PerkinElmer LS55 spectrometer.

4.6.3 Scanning electron microscopy

Particle size and morphology of all dried particles were examined using an Amray 1810T scanning electron microscope (Amray; Bedford, USA) at 20 kV. Prior to the SEM measurement, samples were fixed on aluminium stubs (G301, Plano) with self-adhesive films and spluttered with gold at 20 mA/5 kV (Hummer JR Technics; Munich, Germany) for 1.5 min.

4.6.4 Circular dichroism

CD spectra were recorded on a Jasco J-710 spectropolarimeter (Jasco Deutschland GmbH, Germany) that was constantly purged with nitrogen. Before usage, calibration of the dichrometer was verified using d-10-camphersulfonic acid. HSA samples were prepared equal to FTIR analysis and recorded at a scan speed of 0.20 nm/sec using the Proteus transmission cell described in section 4.5.2. As wavelengths below 185 nm resulted in poor signal-to-noise ratios, spectra ranged between 185 nm and 260 nm. Quantification was performed with the DICHROWEB server [Whitmore et al. 2008] using the SELCON3 analysis program [Sreerama et al. 2000] and SP175 protein reference set from 190 nm - 240 nm [Lees et al. 2006]. For comparison reasons with FTIR data, the numbers for regular and distorted α-helix or β-sheet content were summed up. Validity of evaluation was determined by normalized root mean square deviation (NRMSD) between the measured and calculated data (Equation 4.22).

Equation 4.22
$$NMRSD = \left[\frac{\sum_N \left(\theta_{exptl} - \theta_{calcd}\right)^2}{\sum_N \left(\theta_{exptl}\right)^2} \right]^{1/2}$$

4.6.5 SEC HPLC

The existence of soluble HSA protein aggregates was determined by size exclusion chromatography. The HPLC system consisted of a Prostar 210 solvent delivery systems with two pumps, a Prostar 500 column valve module, a Prostar 325 UV detector and a Model 410 autosampler (Varian Inc., Yarnton, UK). Size exclusion chromatography was performed on a

4.6x250 mm Zorbax GF 250 column (Agilent, West Lothian, UK) with a nominal particle size of 4.0 µm – 4.5 µm and a pore diameter of 150Å. A 20mM phosphate buffer at pH 6.8 with 250 mM NaCl was chosen as mobile phase. The flow rate was constant at 0.250 mL/min under isocratic conditions and the injection volume was 10 µl of a 20 mg/mL HSA solution. Column temperature was 30°C and UV detection of the eluent was carried out at 280 nm. Peak identification and integration was performed using Galaxie chromatography software (Varian Inc, Yarnton, UK).

4.6.6 Homogeneity of liquid feed rate

Liquid feed homogeneity was evaluated at 2 mL/min, 4 mL/min and 6 mL/min for three pump systems exhibiting different levels of pulsation:

- a Microchem rotary pump (KSB AG, Frankenthal, Germany)
- a Pharmacia Biotech P-1 peristaltic pump with 6 rollers (Amersham Pharmacia Biotech Inc., Piscataway, USA)
- an Ismatec ISM597D peristaltic pump with 10 rollers (Ismatec SA, Glattbrugg, Switzerland)

For each pump, a liquid feed rate vs. time profile was recorded with help of a Proline Promass 83A coriolis mass flow unit (Endress+Hause GmbH+Co KG, Weil am Rein, Germany) with and without activated atomization. The output signal of the Promass 83A ranged from 4 to 20 mA for a liquid feed rate between 0 and 10 mL/min and was transformed into a voltage signal between 2 and 10 V by a 500 Ω resistance. This could be recorded by a digital mutlimeter and used to calculate the liquid feed rate by Equation 4.23

Equation 4.23 $$Liquid\ feed\ rate = (x - 2V) \cdot 1{,}25 \frac{ml}{V}$$

where x is the measured voltage.

Data was collected for 10 min after a 5 min equilibrium period to ensure steady state liquid feed rates, while the recording interval was set to 1/s. To be able to describe the extent of fluctuation in liquid feed homogeneity in an objective way, the standard deviations of the individual graphs were calculated.

4.6.7 Particle size distribution

Particle size distributions of the final spray-freeze-dried powders were determined by laser light diffraction using a Malvern Mastersizer S (Malvern Instruments Ltd, Malvern, UK). The instrument was equipped with a 300RF lens with a backscatter detector and a small sample dispersion unit. The final dried product was suspended in acetone at a concentration sufficient to achieve an obscuration between 10-15%. The small volume dispersion unit was set to 2000 rpm. Particle size distribution was calculated as an average of 6 experiments using Mie theory. Refractive indices 1.3590 for acetone and 1.3903 for the sugar matrix were used. The moment diameter of the biggest peak, $d_{v,0.5}$ and the span of the volume distribution were used to characterize the powders. The span is defined by Equation 4.24.

Equation 4.24
$$\text{span} = \frac{d_{v,0.5}}{d_{v,0.9} - d_{v,0.1}}$$

with $d_{v,0.1}$ and $d_{v,0.9}$ describing the particle diameter at 10% and 90% screen underflow.

4.6.8 Infrared imaging

To evaluate the homogeneity of the temperature distribution within the SFD stainless steel containers, infrared images were recorded with a Varioscan 3021 ST IR camera (Infratec GmbH, Dresden, Germany). Images were instantly taken from the top shelf of a Christ Delta 1-24 KD freeze-dryer set to -24°C shelf temperature, after flushing the chamber with nitrogen and removing its lid.

5. FTIR calibration curves

5.1 Introduction

Quantification of protein secondary structure by FTIR analysis can be strongly dependent on subjective factors. Especially evaluation by peak fitting, which can deliver the most detailed information about the conformation of a protein, can easily be biased by incorrect peak placing and false parameters during the iteration process. Other methods, like calculation of the correlation coefficient or area overlap, are more objective but give less information on protein secondary structure (see chapter 3.2).

Therefore, a suitable evaluation method had to be established to ensure objective determination of the changes in protein FTIR spectra during the generation of microparticles. From the approaches commonly applied for quantification of the composition of the amide I band, multivariate data analysis has shown to be the most promising one. It combines a high level of structural information with only few steps of data pre-processing, thus reducing subjectivity [van der Weert et al. 2005]. Initially, a calibration set is generated from the IR spectra of various samples for which the properties of interest, in this work α-helix, as well as intramolecular and intermolecular β-sheet content, have been quantified by other methods. Spectral absorbencies are correlated with the corresponding secondary structure contents by a matrix of absorptivity constants "K" during the calibration step. The structural content of an unknown spectrum can then be quantified with help of K. However, most studies in literature focus on quantification of native proteins and do not show differentiation between native and aggregated conformations [Dousseau et al. 1990; Forato et al. 1998; Wi et al. 1998] which was insufficient for the evaluations performed in this thesis. Therefore a new dataset had to be created with focus on conformations suitable for determining protein damage. As aggregation is often linked with an increase of intermolecular β-sheet at the expense of native structures, such as intramolecular β-sheet and α-helix [Anderle et al. 1987; Carpenter et al. 1998], those structures were included during the generation of datasets for multivariate data analysis.

5.2 Determination of secondary structures for calibration proteins

16 different proteins, showing a wide variety of structural compositions, were dissolved in double distilled and filtered water without further excipients at concentrations between 10 and 20 mg/mL. Spectra were recorded and focused on the non-deconvolved amide I bands and its nearby areas (1800 cm^{-1} – 1580 cm^{-1}). Then, a two point baseline correction was manually performed and the amide I bands were normalized for the same area (Fig. 5.1). In the past, X-ray measurements of pure protein crystals have been frequently employed for the determination of the secondary structure of the calibration proteins [Lee et al. 1990; Rahmelow et al. 1996; Baello et al. 2000]. In this thesis however, secondary structures for the content matrix *C* were determined by peak fitting, offering the following advantages:

- According to Manning [1989], the crystal structure of proteins is not necessarily retained in aqueous solutions. Ca_4-calmodulin and troponin C, for example, exhibited a decrease in helical structures when analyzed in solution [Trewhella et al. 1989].
- By using IR spectra, possible structural changes due to prior processing by the manufacturer, pH-shifts or experimental conditions can be taken into account.
- A discrimination between native and aggregated β-sheets can easily be accomplished during peak fitting while X-ray data often does not discern between those structures [Sreerama et al. 1999].

An increased quantification accuracy was expected if the reference secondary structures for calibration were derived from IR spectra recorded in the liquid state. As peak fitting is a rather subjective quantification method, results were still compared with X-ray data by Levitt [1977], to assure peak assignment and iteration procedures were performed reasonably. The first step during peak fitting consisted of qualitatively detecting the individual peaks adding up to the amide I band using 2nd derivative spectra. Gaussian peaks were placed at the corresponding positions and manually adjusted in width and height until their overall shape roughly matched the amide I band. With help of PeakFit, quantitative evaluation of the secondary structure was performed through an iteration procedure (Fig. 5.2).

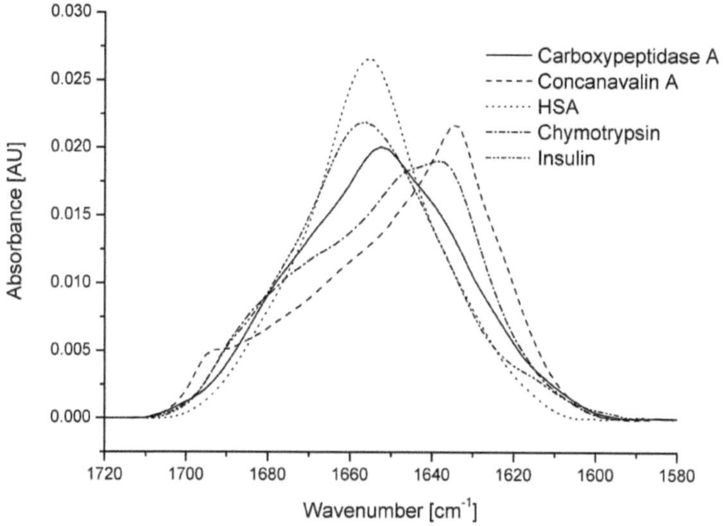

Fig. 5.1: Area normalized amide I bands of five different proteins that were used during calibration. Different secondary structures led to different shapes of the amide I band.

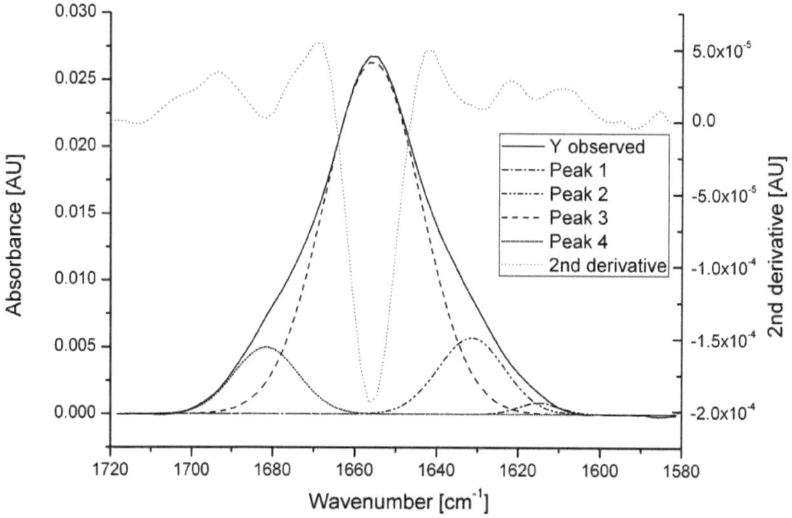

Fig. 5.2: Amide I band peak fit and 2nd derivative spectrum of human serum albumin. The shape of the amide I band is dominated by a strong peak for the α-helix at 1654 cm^{-1}.

Peak positions were fixed while height and width were allowed to vary within five percent. If no solution could be obtained, the initial manual adjustments were altered and iteration was repeated. The fit was considered final as soon as a coefficient of determination $R^2 > 0.999$ was reached. According to literature, peak positions were assigned to individual structural components [Dong et al. 1995; Barth et al. 2002]. As can be seen in Table 5.1, α-helix and unordered structures cannot be discerned in spectra recorded from aqueous solution. Therefore, peaks within those regions were usually assigned to helical components as long as the results were supported by X-ray data. As no satisfactory peak fit could be obtained for α-chymotrypsin, X-ray data was used in this one case only.

Table 5.1: Usual assignment of peak positions to individual secondary structures. Intermolecular β-sheet position was taken from Dong et al. [1995], while other positions were taken from Barth et al. [2002]

Secondary structure	Peak position in H_2O [cm^{-1}]
α-Helix	1648 - 1657
Intramolecular β-sheet	1623 - 1641
Intramolecular β-sheet	1674 – 1695
Intermolecular β-sheet	~ 1616
Turns	1662 – 1686
Disordered	1642 - 1657

5.3 Calibration of the iPLS algorithm

Spectra that were previously used for peak fitting were afterwards implemented as standards for the calibration curve. In this step the shapes and intensities of the area normalized amide I bands were correlated with their percentile secondary structures using an interval partial least squares 1 algorithm [Navea et al. 2005]. During this step, critical shapes ("factors") within the standards were detected and pure component spectra were computed, each one representing only one specific secondary structure (Fig. 5.3). From this point on, the evaluation method was considered calibrated and unknown samples as well as the standards themselves could be quantified. As mentioned in chapter 4.1, secondary structures like β-turn or unordered conformations were not included in the dataset as their influence on an aggregation-focused evaluation was considered negligible. If an excessive number of factors is used for describing a certain secondary structure ("overfitting"), too much information is introduced into the model and overall quantification performance can be reduced [Wi et al. 1998].

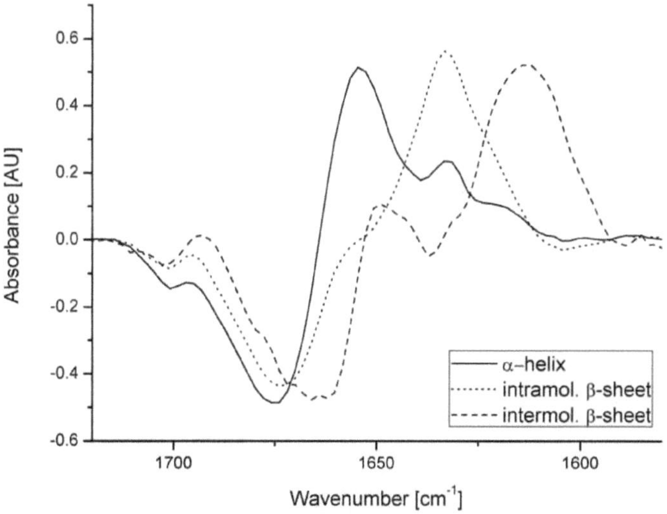

Fig. 5.3: Pure component spectra of critical secondary structures within the amide I band.

To avoid effects due to overfitting, the structural contents of each standard were calculated by cross validation using one, two, three or four factors describing the quantification models. Then, the number of factors giving the lowest predicted residual error sum of squares ("PRESS") was chosen for calibration (see Equation 5.1).

Equation 5.1 $$\sum (y_{iexpd} - y_{ipred})^2$$

where y_{iexp} equals the actual structural content and y_{ipred} the calculated structural content. The ideal number of factors, indicated by the lowest corresponding PRESS values, was two for both α-helix (PRESS=159.80) and intramolecular β-sheet (PRESS=127.92) while one factor was already sufficient for intermolecular β-sheet (PRESS=4.91). The low numbers for intermolecular β-sheet can be explained by its narrow percentile span (0.0% – 9.70%) compared to the other structural components.

Analysis was focused on the following areas to avoid regions containing noise or irrelevant data for the prediction of the individual secondary structures: α-helix 1660 – 1650 cm^{-1}, intramolecular β-sheet 1695 – 1683 cm^{-1} and 1644 – 1620 cm^{-1}, intermolecular β-sheet 1620 – 1595 cm^{-1}. A mean centering technique was applied to the data set before calibration. To evaluate linear relationship, three calibration curves were created from the data sets, one for each type of secondary structure investigated (α-helix, intramolecular β-sheet and intermolecular β-sheet). Calculated secondary structures by multivariate data analysis were plotted against structural contents as determined by peak fitting ("actual") (Fig. 5.4). As shown in Table 5.2, the calculated α-helix content ranged from 0% (concanavalin A) to 78.04% (myoglobin). Insulin showed highest deviation from actual α-helical values (56.14% actual vs. 51.23% calculated). As mentioned earlier, structural contents of α-chymotrypsin could not be specified by peak fitting due to problems during peak assignment and thus were replaced by values determined by X-ray analysis. Values calculated for intramolecular β-sheet ranged from 10.76% (HSA) to 63.89% (concanavalin A). No calculated result was more than 3.69% away from its actual value (e.g. concanavalin A). The data set for intermolecular β-sheet only ranged from 0.23% (glucagon) to 9.70% (concanavalin A). Even though most protein standards were pre-lyophilized by the supplier, no extensive damage to secondary structure was induced which explains the low intermolecular β-sheet contents. As X-ray analysis did not discern between intra- and intermolecular β-sheets, values taken for α-chymotrypsin were assigned to intramolecular β-sheet only. β-Galactosidase showed the highest deviation between actual and calculated values (1.09%).

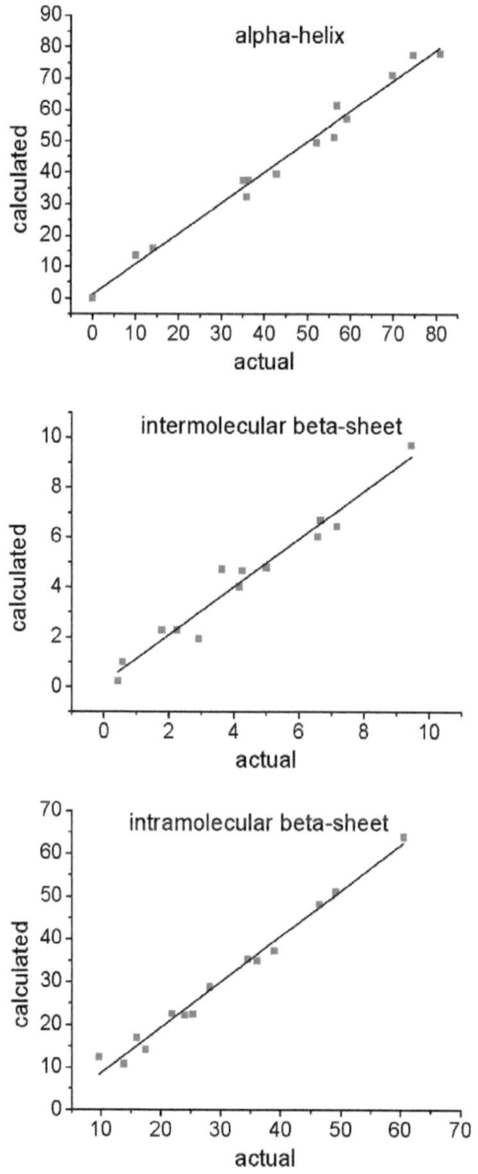

Fig. 5.4: Calibration curves created from the data sets. A linear relationship represents good agreement between actual and calculated structural content.

Table 5.2: Comparison of the secondary structure by peak fitting (actual) with calculated values (calculated).

Protein	α-Helix (actual)	α-Helix (calculated)	Intramol. β -sheet (actual)	Intramol. β-sheet (calculated)	Intermol. β -sheet (actual)	Intermol. β-sheet (calculated)
Alkaline phosphatase	36.21%	37.68%	34.49%	35.15%	4.26%	4.66%
Bovine serum albumin	69.64%	71.19%	17.39%	13.95%	1.78%	2.28%
Carbonic anhydrase	14.05%	15.99%	46.29%	47.59%	7.15%	6.44%
Carboxypeptidase A	35.04%	37.45%	28.18%	27.74%	6.56%	6.03%
Catalase	35.86%	32.32%	38.91%	36.55%	6.64%	6.69%
Concanavalin A	0.00%	0.00%	60.45%	63.89%	9.45%	9.70%
α-Chymotrypsin	10.00%	13.61%	49.00%	52.47%	n/a	5.59%
β-Galactosidase	42.78%	39.51%	36.05%	35.47%	3.63%	4.72%
Glucagon	59.12%	57.15%	15.88%	17.05%	0.42%	0.23%
Haemoglobin	74.68%	79.59%	10.63%	10.64%	2.79%	2.09%
Human serum albumin	74.48%	77.62%	13.81%	10.76%	0.57%	1.00%
Insulin	56.14%	51.23%	23.92%	22.46%	5.00%	4.79%
Lactic dehydrogenase	56.81%	61.39%	25.32%	23.46%	2.92%	1.94%
Lysozyme	51.92%	49.57%	21.84%	21.84%	4.17%	4.03%
Myoglobin	80.71%	78.04%	9.68%	12.56%	2.25%	2.28%
Ribonuclease A	24.78%	23.39%	40.26%	42.09%	2.92%	3.65%

The correlation coefficient r (Equation 5.2) was used to quantify the linear relationship between actual and calculated values. Results lay between 0.992 for α-helix and intramolecular β-sheet and 0.979 for intermolecular β-sheet, indicating strong linear correlations.

Equation 5.2
$$r = \frac{n\sum x_i y_i - \sum x_i \sum y_i}{\sqrt{n\sum x_i^2 - (\sum x_i)^2}\sqrt{n\sum y_i^2 - (\sum y_i)^2}}$$

where n equals the number of standards and x_i and y_i the actual and calculated values.

The uncertainty of the calibration model was evaluated by root mean square error (RMSE) of the calibration curves (Equation 5.3). Values for α-helix, intramolecular β-sheet and intermolecular β-sheet were 2.95, 2.24 and 0.53 respectively.

Equation 5.3
$$RMSE = \sqrt{\frac{\sum (x_i - y_i)^2}{n}}$$

where n equals the number of standards and x_i and y_i the actual and calculated values.

Validity of results was evaluated by including two more standards for validation purposes, hemoglobin for highly helical, and ribonuclease A for β-sheet rich proteins. Secondary structures were again determined by peak fitting and compared to the calculated values. However, validation standards were not included in the calibration set and did not affect its compilation. A performance index, calculated as the RMSE, for the validation standards was calculated giving information on how well unknown samples are quantified. Results were 0.986, 0.144 and 0.495 for α-helix, intramolecular β-sheet and intermolecular β-sheet respectively, indicating good quantification performance.

To minimize any bias by outliers, a cross validation was performed. Each calibration standard was quantified as if it were a validation standard. This was accomplished by sequentially removing one standard from the calibration set, calibrating the method and using the new calibration model to quantify the excluded standard. The software repeated the process until all the calibration standards were quantified as validation standards. Correlation coefficients r for α-helix, intramolecular β-sheet and intermolecular β-sheet were 0.990, 0.982 and 0.972 while RMSE of cross validation was 3.38, 3.02 and 0.615, respectively. Based on these results no protein was considered an outlier and had to be removed from the calibration step.

Comparing the calculated results with literature showed good agreement for most of the included proteins (Table 5.3). Only β-sheet content of myoglobin and haemoglobin were significantly higher than values determined by X-ray (by 12% and 10% respectively). As both proteins exhibit a combination of very high α-helix and low β-sheet content, results could be biased by the strong absorbance between 1660 cm^{-1} and 1650 cm^{-1}, influencing the adjacent region actually assigned to β-sheet. Additionally, changes to secondary structure during crystallization cannot be ruled out completely [Manning 1989] (see chapter 5.2).

Table 5.3: Comparison of secondary structures as found by Levitt with calculated data, presented in this work [Levitt et al. 1977].

Protein	α-Helix (X-ray)	α-Helix (FTIR)	β -Sheet (X-ray)	Intramol. β-sheet (FTIR)
Carbonic anhydrase	16%	16%	45%	48%
Carboxy-peptidase A	39%	38%	30%	29%
Concanavalin A	3%	0%	60%	64%
α-Chymotrypsin	10%	14%	49%	51%
Haemoglobin	86%	80%	0%	10%
Insulin	53%	51%	15%	22%
Lysozyme	46%	50%	19%	22%
Myoglobin	85%	78%	0%	12%
Ribonuclease A	23%	23%	46%	42%

5.4 Validation of the quantification procedure

5.4.1 Bias due to baseline effects

The Proteus transmission cell uses very thin silicon spacers (d=0.6 μm) to compensate for the strong absorbance of water between 1700 cm^{-1} and 1600 cm^{-1}. Therefore, small deviations in pathlength between sample and background measurements can lead to substantial changes in absorbance possibly affecting the shape of the amide I band. Fig. 5.5 shows the relation between the protein spectra of a-CT and HSA recorded at 10 mg/mL and six different blank spectra, each one immediately taken after the background was recorded. As can be seen, water absorbance constituted a considerable part of the amide I band at the given concentration and could augment or lower its intensity. This presents a bias due to limitations by the FTIR spectrometer instrumentation, not by the iPLS algorithm itself, and might negatively affect the precision of quantification. However, no information on standard deviations was available as the recorded amide I bands consisted of averaged scans to reduce spectral noise. Therefore, the influence of baseline fluctuations on the evaluation of protein secondary structure had to be evaluated separately.

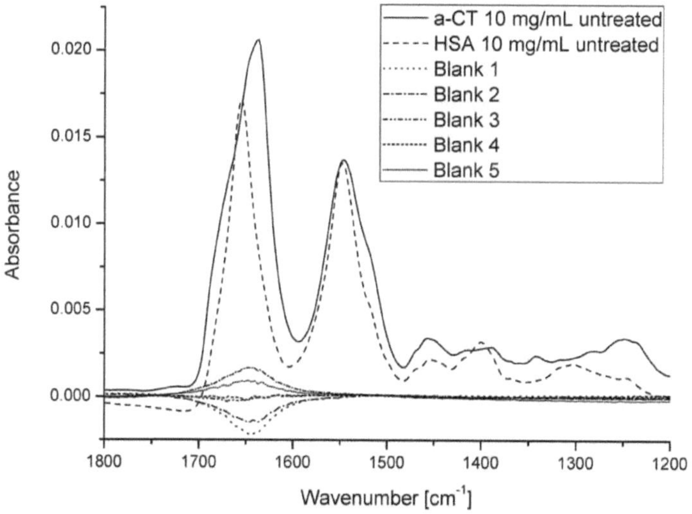

Fig. 5.5: FTIR absorbance spectra of a-CT and HSA at concentrations of 10 mg/mL as well as six individually recorded blank spectra.

The blank spectra presented in Fig. 5.5 were added to different a-CT and HSA protein spectra, previously recorded at concentrations of 5, 10, 30 and 100 mg/mL respectively. This made possible baseline fluctuations between individual measurements visible.

Table 5.4 displays the mean and standard deviation (sdv) values calculated for the secondary structures of a-CT. Absorbance of the 5 mg/mL solution was very weak (around 0.008) making the signal susceptible to baseline effects. This is visible from the high standard deviations up to 2.5% for intramolecular β-sheet. In this case, subtle damage to secondary structure could not be quantified as changes within the amide I band could not be discerned from noise. By doubling the concentration, precision of quantification increased substantially leading to sdv values between 0.3% and 0.6%. Even higher concentrations further reduced deviations during the measurements, but to a smaller extent.

Measurements were performed accordingly for HSA. The 5 mg/mL solution gave an inadequate signal to noise ratio leading to a sdv up 10.88% for α-helix. By doubling the concentration the precision of quantification could be improved substantially (Table 5.5): The sdv values for α-helix and intramolecular β-sheet dropped to 2.8% and 2.2% respectively. Further increases in concentration consecutively improved the accuracy. However, the achieved sdvs always lay above the values determined for a-CT indicating inferior overall evaluation performance for HSA.

The question still remained why HSA showed a higher uncertainty of quantification than a-CT at equal concentrations. The most plausible reason would be that the shape of the amide I band differed clearly for both proteins. First, the maximum of HSA coincided with the maxima/minima of the blank samples, making it more susceptible to fluctuations (see Fig. 5.5). Second, the band exhibited a high height-to-width ratio resulting in a rather sharp peak. Therefore, any fluctuation led to more severe consequences for HSA than for a-CT because its amide I band comprised of several overlapping peaks.

Surprisingly, higher concentrations seemed to promote changes to protein secondary structure. In case of a-CT, mean values for α-helix were reduced from 15% (10 mg/mL) to 13.1% (100 mg/mL) while intermolecular β-sheet rose from 5.4% to 6.3%. Over the same concentrations, HSA showed a reduction in helical structures as well (down by 1.3%) accompanied by increases in intramolecular β-sheet (up by 1.2%). This way, advantages of the high signal-to-noise ratio at elevated concentrations were partially diminished due to changes in protein secondary structure. 100 mg/mL a-CT and HSA solutions also showed inferior handling properties because viscosity increased substantially. This reduced their applicability for FTIR analysis as the danger of clogging the measurement cell increased noticeably. As a consequence, protein concentrations between 10 and 30 mg/mL were used in the following chapters for recording FTIR spectra from aqueous protein solutions.

Table 5.4: Precision of the quantification of a-CT secondary structure depending on the sample concentration.

	5 mg/mL a-CT		**10 mg/mL a-CT**		**30 mg/mL a-CT**		**100 mg/mL a-CT**	
	mean	sdv	mean	sdv	mean	sdv	mean	sdv
α-Helix	14.5%	1.2%	15.0%	0.3%	14.0%	0.2%	13.1%	0.1%
Intramol. β-sheet	52.1%	2.5%	50.3%	0.6%	50.9%	0.4%	50.5%	0.1%
Intermol. β-sheet	5.0%	1.4%	5.4%	0.4%	5.6%	0.2%	6.3%	0.1%

Table 5.5: Precision of the quantification of HSA secondary structure at different sample concentrations.

	5 mg/mL HSA		**10 mg/mL HSA**		**30 mg/mL HSA**		**100 mg/mL HSA**	
	mean	sdv	mean	sdv	mean	sdv	mean	sdv
α-Helix	80.9%	10.9%	78.3%	2.8%	77.1%	2.0%	77.0%	0.5%
Intramol. β-sheet	9.0%	6.1%	9.7%	2.2%	10.3%	1.2%	10.9%	0.3%
Intermol. β-sheet	1.2%	1.0%	1.0%	0.6%	1.4%	0.3%	1.3%	0.1%

To further evaluate the applicability and precision of the iPLS algorithm, changes in the secondary structure of glucagon and HSA were quantified using the calibration curves. Results were then compared with secondary structure analysis performed by CD and peak fitting. In case of HSA, aggregation behavior was additionally determined by size exclusion chromatography and turbidity analysis.

5.4.2 Heat denaturation of human serum albumin

According to literature, denaturation temperature of HSA lies between 60°C and 65°C depending on the actual pH [Barone 1992]. Measurement of a freshly dissolved pure protein solution indicated a pH of 7.05 at 25°C, and therefore a denaturation temperature of 65°C was expected. HSA solutions with a concentration of 20 mg/mL were exposed to temperatures of 25°C, 40°C, 60°C, 70°C and 80°C for 30 min in a waterbath. After cooling down to room temperature, the samples were centrifuged and subsequently analyzed. As can be seen in Table 5.6, native structure of HSA, determined by iPLS, underwent only minor changes until 60°C. In comparison to the sample kept at 25°C, helical structures were reduced by 5.71% while intra- and intermolecular β-sheets gained 3.2% and 0.84%, respectively.

Table 5.6: Changes in secondary structure of HSA due to elevated temperatures.

Temperature	Method	α-Helix	Intramol. β-sheet	Intermol. β-sheet
25°C	iPLS	77.62%	10.76%	1.00%
	Peak Fit	76.23%	12.58%	1.18%
	CD	67.1%	3.5%	
40°C	iPLS	74.74%	12.50%	1.50%
	Peak Fit	75.51%	13.19%	1.14%
	CD	64.1%	4.5%	
60°C	iPLS	71.91%	13.96%	1.84%
	Peak Fit	72.59%	13.52%	2.03%
	CD	62.1%	5.2%	
70°C	iPLS	54.14%	22.05%	6.38%
	Peak Fit	59.83%	20.04%	6.25%
	CD	51.5%	12.5%	
80°C	iPLS	36.69%	29.52%	11.52%
	Peak Fit	45.61%	27.96%	11.36%
	CD	41.3%	22.4%	

The remaining 1.67% were distributed between β-turn and unordered structures. Any further increase in temperature led to a strong decrease of α-helix (down to 36.69%) and to an increase in intramolecular and intermolecular β-sheet (up to 29.52% and 11.52% respectively), supporting the DSC results by Barone [1992]. Peak fitting was applied to verify results obtained by the calibration curves using exactly the same amide I bands as for the quantification by the iPLS algorithm. For 25°C to 60°C results showed very good agreement between the two techniques, only exhibiting fluctuations within 2%. For higher temperatures differences increased up to 8.92% for α-helix at 80°C. The trend to lower helical values by the calibration curve at 70°C and 80°C can be explained by two observations: First, the spectral region for α-helix is only 10 wavenumbers wide (from 1660 cm^{-1} – 1650 cm^{-1}) leaving a narrow window for quantification. As denaturation of HSA is linked with an overall broadening of the amide I band (Fig. 5.6) spectral features related to α-helix could shift beyond the limits set by calibration, thereby avoiding detection. Second, the shape of the amide I band changed substantially during heating, matching no standard defined during calibration. This could have additionally increased the error of quantification.

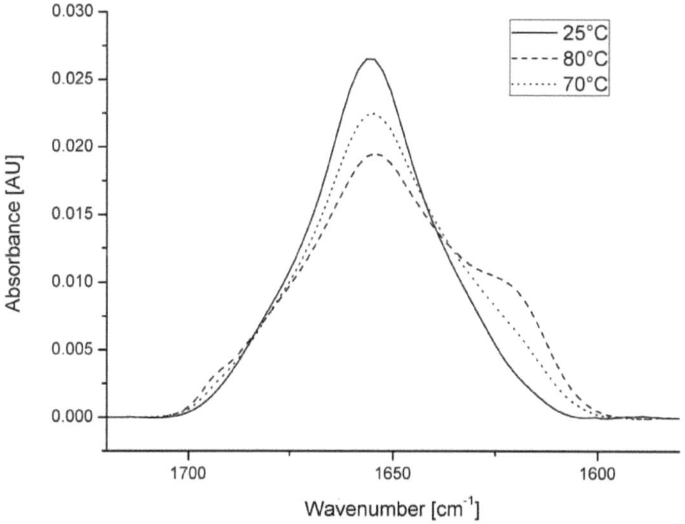

Fig. 5.6: Changes of the amide I band of HSA after heat treatment. The spectrum showed a decrease in height and spectral broadening. The shoulder at 1618 cm^{-1} correlates with intermolecular β-sheet due to newly formed aggregates.

For further validation, data obtained by FTIR spectroscopy was compared to the results from CD measurements (see Table 5.6). As evaluation by CD could not discern between intramolecular and intermolecular conformations, only one value is available for the β-sheet content. However, the tendency for the increase in formation of the β-sheet content at the expense of the α-helix content was still visible. Freshly dissolved HSA showed a secondary structure of mainly α-helix (67.1%) and only very little β-sheet (3.5%). In analogy to FTIR measurements, only minor changes occurred until 60°C, resulting in a small decline in α-helix by 5.0% and slight increase in β-sheet content by 1.7%. Increasing temperatures to 70°C and 80°C, however, inflicted strong protein damage (Fig. 5.7): The helical content was reduced by 25.8%, and β-sheet increased by 18.9% compared to its original values. The NRMSD of all evaluations, describing the precision of quantification, stayed below 0.1, indicating good fitting except for HSA at 80°C (0.146) which was still considered acceptable.

In comparison to FTIR, results from CD gave lower absolute values for helical (up to 10.52% at 25°C) and β-sheet content (up to 18.64% at 80°C).

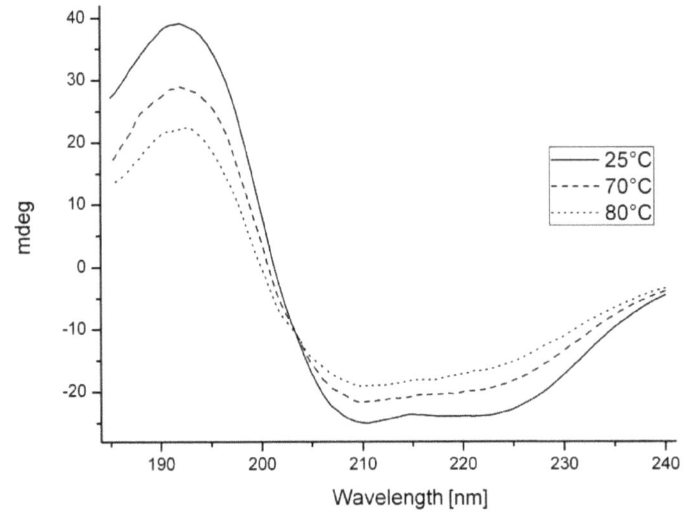

Fig. 5.7: Circular dichroism spectra of HSA. Heat treatment led to a decrease of native conformations and to an increase in β-sheet and unordered conformations.

This is not surprising as systematic deviations between both techniques have been previously reported in literature [Susi et al. 1985]. In this case, the most plausible explanation is that different references were used for calibration of the datasets. The SP175 dataset was created from X-ray structures using the DSSP algorithm [Lees et al. 2006] while the FTIR dataset was created by peak fitting of infrared spectra and validated with X-ray data created by Levitt [1977]. However, both methods showed that about 72% of the loss in α-helix could be associated with an increase in β-sheet during denaturation. Therefore, the α-β transition seems to be a feasible way for quantifying protein damage.

HSA is known to form soluble aggregates during storage at elevated temperatures. Solubility decreases with increasing aggregate size finally leading to protein precipitation [Wang 2005]. To determine a possible correlation between the formation of soluble aggregates and an increase in intermolecular β-sheet during heating, samples were additionally analyzed by size exclusion chromatography (SEC). Until 60°C only one monomer peak was detectable in the chromatogram at an elution time of 10 mins.

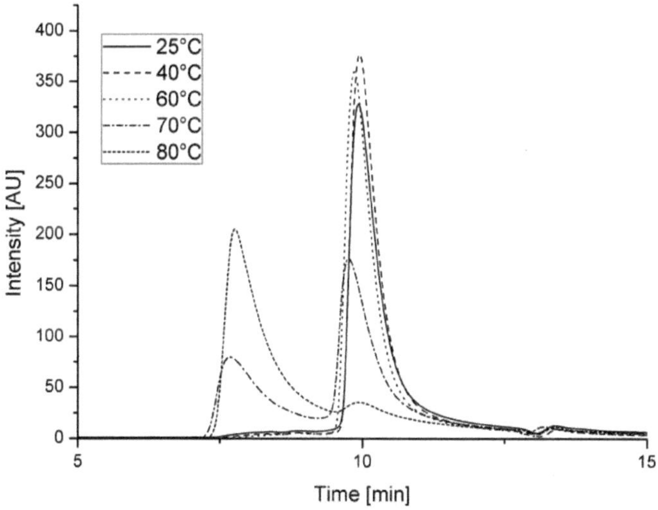

Fig. 5.8: SEC diagram of heat treated HSA. Monomer content (detectable at 10 mins) stayed constant until 60°C with no aggregate peak visible. At 70°C and 80°C noticeable aggregate formation occurred (signal after 7 – 8 min).

Increasing the temperature to 70°C decreased the height of the monomer peak and gave rise to a new signal at 8 minutes which could be assigned to aggregated HSA molecules (Fig. 5.8). At 80°C, aggregates increased strongly at the expense of monomers. These results were in good agreement to the findings from FTIR and CD analysis in the paragraphs above.

Finally, turbidity analysis at 350 nm for the detection of soluble and insoluble aggregates supported the results determined by HPLC. For 25°C, 40°C and 60°C, transmission lay between 0.730 (rel. sdv=0.21%) and 0.721 (rel. sdv=0.08%), indicating only minor formation of aggregates. However, at 70°C and 80°C transmission experienced a strong decrease down to 0.659 (rel. sdv=0.26%) and 0.646 (rel.sdv= 0.39%), respectively, which is once again in concurrence with the results presented earlier. The noticeable changes in transmission were accompanied by precipitation of HSA.

In summary, all HSA evaluations supported the approach performed in this thesis to quantify protein damage by measuring the transition from native structures to intermolecular (and partially intramolecular) β-sheet.

5.4.3 Fibrillation of Glucagon

Glucagon is a 29 amino acid polypeptide that is known to fibrillate in solution at high concentrations and acidic pH [Onoue et al. 2004]. Depending on protein concentration and polarity of the solvent, freshly dissolved glucagon can form a predominantly helical or random coil structure that transforms completely into β-sheets during fibrillation [Moran et al. 1977; Onoue et al. 2006]. For fibrillation analysis, glucagon solutions (7 mg/mL in AcOH) were kept at room temperature and stirred constantly. Samples were taken at 1h intervals and subsequently analyzed after centrifugation. Immediately after dissolving in 1% AcOH, the FTIR spectrum of Glucagon showed a maximum at 1656 cm^{-1} typical for high α-helix content. Within 4h the spectrum underwent substantial changes giving rise to two new peaks at 1630 cm^{-1} and 1614 cm^{-1}, assigned to intra- and intermolecular β-sheets (Fig. 5.9). Quantification by peak fitting showed that native α-helix dropped quickly from 64.82% to 0% after only 4h. In the same time intramolecular β-sheet increased from 14.36% to 34.99% and intermolecular β-sheet 0.42% to 16.92%. The remaining 27.69% of the former α-helix were split up between an increase of unordered conformations and β-turns. Quantification by iPLS showed an even higher α-β transition.

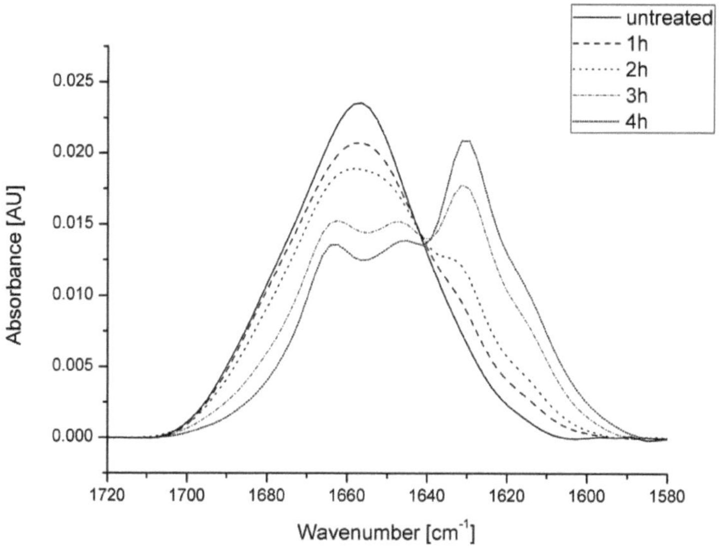

Fig. 5.9: FTIR spectra of glucagon. During fibrillation the maximum for α-helix completely vanished. Two new peaks were formed at 1630 cm^{-1} and 1614 cm^{-1} typical for intra- and intermolecular β-sheet.

α-Helix content dropped from 60.57% to 0% within 4h while intramolecular and intermolecular β-sheets rose from 15.88% to 40.53% and 0.33% to 21.96%, respectively. As with HSA, 76% of the loss in helical structures could be attributed to the formation of β-sheets. Those results were in good agreement with the CD results from Moran, claiming that glucagon at high concentrations assumes a predominantly α-helical structure (48%) that devolves into β-sheet (54%) during aging [Moran et al. 1977]. As no sufficient signal-to-noise ratio could be obtained from CD setup used in this work, the FTIR results could only be compared to literature.

5.5 Overall comparison and discussion

Statistical validation of the calibration curves as well as comparison with X-ray data supported the reliability of evaluation by iPLS algorithm. The calculated results were reproducible and minimized any influence by the user, thus making quantification by FTIR spectroscopy much more objective than peak fitting. Furthermore, quantification could be performed quickly as the only processing steps after recording the spectrum consisted of baseline correction and area normalization. Analysis of baseline effects indicated that spectra should be taken at concentrations of 10 mg/mL or higher due to limitations of the FTIR cuvette used. The usage of different cuvettes or detectors could even make the quantification of lower concentrated samples possible.

Comparison of the FTIR results of HSA and glucagon with CD showed minor differences between the two methods of analysis. As stated in chapter 5.4.2, this was not surprising as different datasets have been used for calibrating both methods. Of course, one must keep in mind that possible errors were willingly tolerated during quantification of the calibration standards by peak fitting. But more importantly, the method developed in this thesis was aimed at objectively quantifying changes to secondary structure, not at determining the absolute values. At this point CD and FTIR concurred indicating that roughly 70% of native secondary structure is transformed into intermolecular (and partially intramolecular) β-sheet during denaturation of the investigated proteins.

Finally, it was possible to link aggregate formation of HSA detected by SEC-HPLC and turbidity analysis to the formation of inter- and intramolecular β-sheets. This means that shifts from native structure to β-sheets should be useable for quantifying damage to protein secondary structure and possible aggregate formation.

The data set used during calibration consisted of proteins in their native states. Therefore, the calibration curve for intermolecular β-sheet did not include values higher than 10%. By including denatured proteins as standards, quantification reliability could be improved even further. In addition, the iPLS algorithm should be able to determine protein secondary structure from solid samples as well because position of the individual peaks within the amide I band remains generally the same. However, shifts to lower wavenumbers are possible in the solid state. Therefore, the validity of quantification procedure must be assessed prior to applying the calibration curves on solid samples. This would greatly increase the field of application of this evaluation method.

6. Preparation of pure protein microparticles by spray-freeze-drying

6.1 Introduction

Microparticles consisting of a-CT or HSA at concentrations of 10 mg/mL and 100 mg/mL were generated by SFD without any excipients. The impact of different nozzle types (four ultrasonic nozzle at operating frequencies of 25 kHz, 48 kHz, 60 kHz, 120 kHz and one two-fluid nozzle with a cap orifice of 0.7 mm) on protein stability as well as particle appearance was evaluated. The whole process of spray-freeze-drying, consisting of

- atomization
- atomization and freezing
- the complete SFD process

was split up into its individual preparation steps to gain further insight into the procedure and delineate separate effects. The standard procedure up-to-date was to spray the protein solution into stainless steel pans filled with cryogen, that also served as bulk containers during the following freeze-drying step [Sonner 2002; Maa et al. 2004; van Drooge et al. 2005]. In this thesis, however, the frozen particles were lyophilized using 20 cc freeze-drying vials, as explained in chapter 4.3.1. By using only these well established freeze-drying containers, the heat transfer between shelf and product is facilitated which improves reproducibility [Costantino et al. 2004]. Another problem when utilizing stainless steel pans is shown in Fig. 6.1. The inhomogeneity of the heat distribution throughout the container is obvious, exhibiting a temperature difference between 5°C and 10°C. At this time any ice inside the pan has already been removed. If ice was still present, temperature differences were presumably even higher due to continuous sublimation [Costantino et al. 2004]. Hence, the use of standard FD-vials should lead to more representative results during spray-freeze-drying.

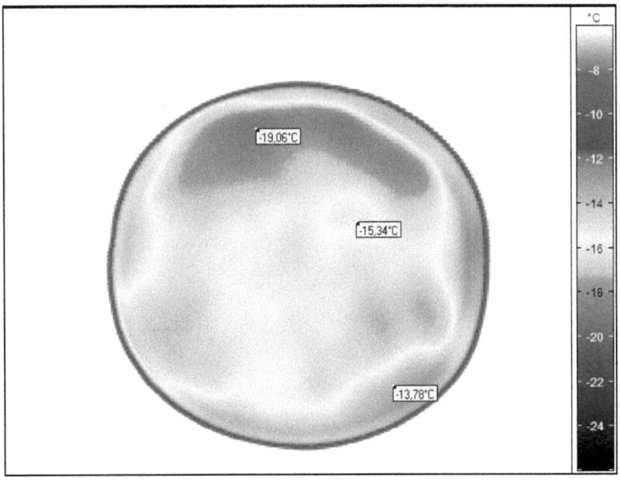

Fig. 6.1: Differences in temperature distribution inside a stainless-steel bowl after 45 min of primary drying. The shelf temperature during this step was set to -24°C.

The individual SFD preparation steps were investigated in the following ways:

- *Liquid Atomization*

  The liquid feed was sprayed directly into a beaker and subsequently analyzed.

- *Freezing and subsequent thawing at room temperature*

  Those experiments were performed equal to the complete SFD process, but without the final freeze-drying step. Instead, the vials were stoppered after all of the LN_2 had boiled off and the frozen particles were allowed to thaw at room temperature.

- *Complete SFD process*

  Powder particles were reconstituted in double-distilled and filtered water at the desired concentrations and then analyzed.

To evaluate the correlation between concentration and protein damage, all three evaluation methods were conducted with 10 mg/mL and 100 mg/mL protein solutions. Throughout the experiments, a liquid flow rate of 1 mL/min and an atomizing power input of 3W were used to achieve comparable settings for all ultrasonic nozzles. The very low liquid flow rate was chosen, because Sonner [2002] determined reduced pulsation effects of the liquid feed for lower peristaltic pump speeds, thus resulting in a narrower droplet size distribution.

According to Sono-Tek [2009], mean number droplet sizes between 18 μm (120 kHz) and 65 μm (25 kHz) can be generated by ultrasound atomization, with higher nozzle frequencies producing lower droplet diameters (values determined for pure water). For two-fluid atomization however, droplet sizes are dependent on atomizing air-flow and liquid feed rates. A low atomizing air-flow in combination with a high liquid feed rate favors the generation of larger droplets [Maa et al. 1999; Maury et al. 2005]. Therefore, the two-fluid nozzle had to be operated at different feed rates than the ultrasound nozzles to achieve comparable droplet sizes. Throughout the atomization experiments, air-flow rate was set to 550 Nl/h (normlitres per hour) while pump speed was set to 10 mL/min. For solutions, the droplet sizes will differ, as other factors like surface tension, viscosity and the density of the liquid feed also affect the droplet diameter [Masters 1991].

For each step, protein secondary and tertiary structures were evaluated by FTIR and fluorescence spectroscopy. Shape and appearance of the SFD products were also compared using SEM. For a-CT, overall enzyme stability was additionally determined by UV/Vis spectroscopic activity assay.

6.2 α-Chymotrypsin particles from low concentrated solutions (10 mg/mL)

6.2.1 Atomization experiments

Atomization of the low concentrated α-chymotrypsin solution induced only subtle damage to the protein. a-CT structure contains 8 tryptophan residues [Desie et al. 1986] that, upon excitation at 295 nm, give rise to a fluorescence emission maximum at ~342 nm in aqueous solutions. If tryptophan is repositioned from the rather hydrophobic interior to the periphery of the protein (as is the case during denaturation), a bathochrome shift in fluorescence emission maximum is observed [Vivian et al. 2001]. As can be seen in Fig. 6.2a, fluorescence maxima showed a small redshift after atomization in comparison to λ_{max} of the untreated protein (341.5 nm). Maxima of the atomized samples lay between 342.1 nm and and 342.3 nm for all nozzles evaluated, except for the 25 kHz design which led to a bathochrome shift to 343.7 nm. Therefore, it seems that a-CT tertiary structure was little affected during atomization. Only the 25 kHz nozzle induced noticeable damage to the protein tertiary structure, visible by the comparably large redshift.

In analogy to fluorescence spectroscopy, FTIR analysis showed only little damage of a-CT secondary structure (Fig. 6.2b). For most of the atomization experiments, changes to native structures (15.0% α-helix, 50.5% intramolecular β-sheet, 5.3% intermolecular β-sheet) were within the margin of error determined in chapter 5.4.1. However, a trend to reduced helical and intramolecular as well as increased intermolecular content was visible, suggesting marginal aggregate formation (Fig. 6.2c). Highest damage was caused by the 25 kHz nozzle which increased intermolecular β-sheet by 1.5%, while the other nozzles showed increases by values between 0.7% and 1.3% (see Table 6.1).

Enzyme activity assay indicated slight reductions in overall a-CT stability by the atomization step. Compared to the freshly dissolved protein, activity dropped noticeably to 88.8% after atomizing with the 25 kHz nozzle. On the other hand, spraying at higher frequencies led to residual activities between 93.3% and 96.5% suggesting only subtle protein damage (Fig. 6.2d). Atomization with the two-fluid nozzle design led to results comparable to the 25 kHz nozzle. In spite of the high standard deviation (sdv=7%), this is still surprising considering the low damage detected for secondary and tertiary structure.

An additional indicator for elevated protein stress during atomization at 25 kHz was the formation of foam that was visible directly after the spraying step. Neither the two-fluid nor the other ultrasound nozzles had a comparable effect on the a-CT solutions. Considering the entire SFD process, atomization of the low concentrated chymotrypsin solution seemed to have negligible effect on protein stability - except for the 25 kHz nozzle.

Table 6.1: Changes to protein secondary structure (concentration 10 mg/mL) caused by the atomization step.

Nozzle type	α-Helix	Intramol. β-sheet	Intermol. β-sheet
25 kHz nozzle	-0.3%	-1.0%	+1.5%
48 kHz nozzle	-0.3%	-0.4%	+1.3%
60 kHz nozzle	-0.3%	-0.1%	+1.0%
120 kHz nozzle	-0.2%	-0.3%	+1.2%
Two-fluid nozzle	-0.1%	-0.2%	+0.7%

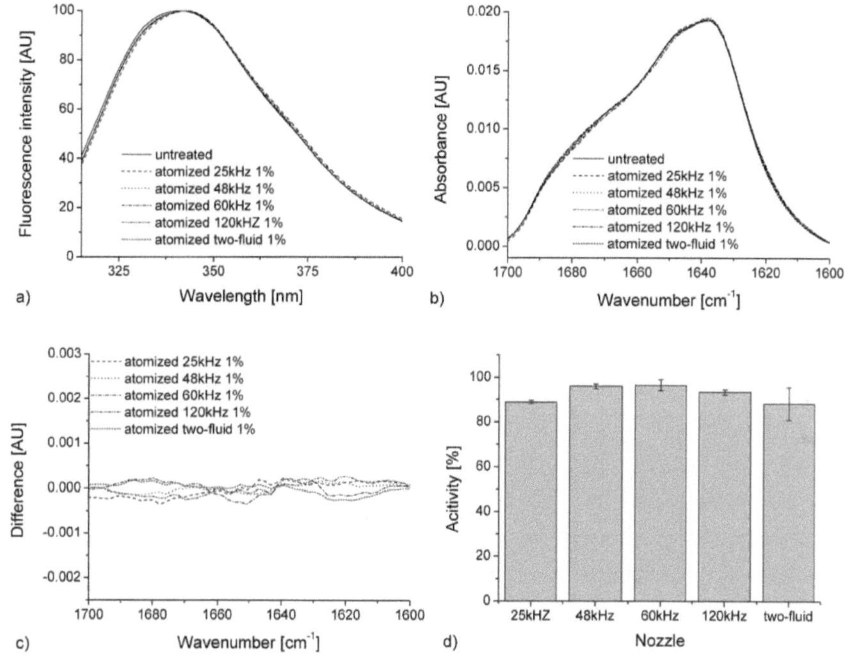

Fig. 6.2: Atomization experiments performed using a 10 mg/mL a-CT solution without any excipients. a) Tryptophan fluorescence spectra, b) FTIR amide I bands, c) FTIR difference spectra of the atomized and untreated samples, d) a-CT activity assays.

6.2.2 Freeze-thaw experiments

The ultrasonic nozzles proved to be very well suited for the freeze-thaw experiments. After atomization, the fine droplet spray softly descended into the cryogen and was immediately frozen. Smaller particles instantly sank into the LN_2, while the larger ones stayed shortly at the surface before sinking as well. This was caused by the small heat of vaporization of nitrogen, leading to an insulating gaseous layer between the particles and the cryogen known as the Leidenfrost effect [Engstrom et al. 2007]. Ice exhibits a higher density than LN_2 (917 kg/m^3 vs. 808 kg/m^3), so the frozen particles could easily be gathered at the bottom of the bowl containing the cryogen and filled into the freeze-drying vials through a gauge. Utilization of the two-fluid nozzle during the freeze-thaw experiments was not possible, as the high atomization air-flow and liquid feed rate of the nozzle gave rise to strong boiling of the LN_2. Inherent with the agitation of the LN_2 was a further increase in product blow out as described earlier by Sonner [2002] resulting in very low product yields. Therefore, no numbers can be displayed for the freeze-thaw experiments using a two-fluid nozzle.

Analysis of the low concentrated a-CT solutions after freezing and subsequent thawing yielded slightly superior results compared to atomization alone. Fluorescence spectra showed minor redshifts from 341.5 nm to wavelengths between 342.3 nm (60 kHz) and 342.7 nm (25 kHz) (Fig. 6.3a). Surprisingly, damage to tertiary structure by the 25 kHz nozzle design was reduced by a small amount while the other bathochrome shifts lay roughly within the region determined during the atomization experiments.

Formation of aggregates during atomization, detected by a slight increase in intermolecular β-sheet, could be completely reversed by quench freezing. Aggregates seem to have been reorganized in intramolecular β-sheet which increased by values between 0.4% and 1.0% for the 48 kHz, 60 kHz and 120 kHz nozzles (Table 6.2). Even any damage induced by the 25 kHz nozzle design was completely prevented by immediate freezing. This observation was also macroscopically detectable in Fig. 6.3b+c by the increase in absorbance between 1690 cm^{-1} and 1660 cm^{-1} which corresponds to a mixture of intramolecular β-sheets and β-turns.

Enzyme activity assay also suggested a recovery in overall enzyme stability. Freeze-thaw experiments using the 25 kHz nozzle exhibited an increase in activity by 4.6% compared to atomization alone. At higher nozzle frequencies, stability could even be completely preserved resulting in residual a-CT activities between 97.4% and 100% (Fig. 6.3d). Hence, atomization followed by instant quench freezing did not affect a-CT stability at low concentrations.

Table 6.2: The effect of freezing and subsequent thawing on a-CT secondary structure (10 mg/mL).

Nozzle type	α-Helix	Intramol. β-sheet	Intermol. β-sheet
25 kHz nozzle	-0.3%	±0.2%	±0.0%
48 kHz nozzle	-0.6%	+0.4%	±0.0%
60 kHz nozzle	-0.4%	+0.6%	±0.0%
120 kHz nozzle	-0.7%	+1.0%	-0.3%

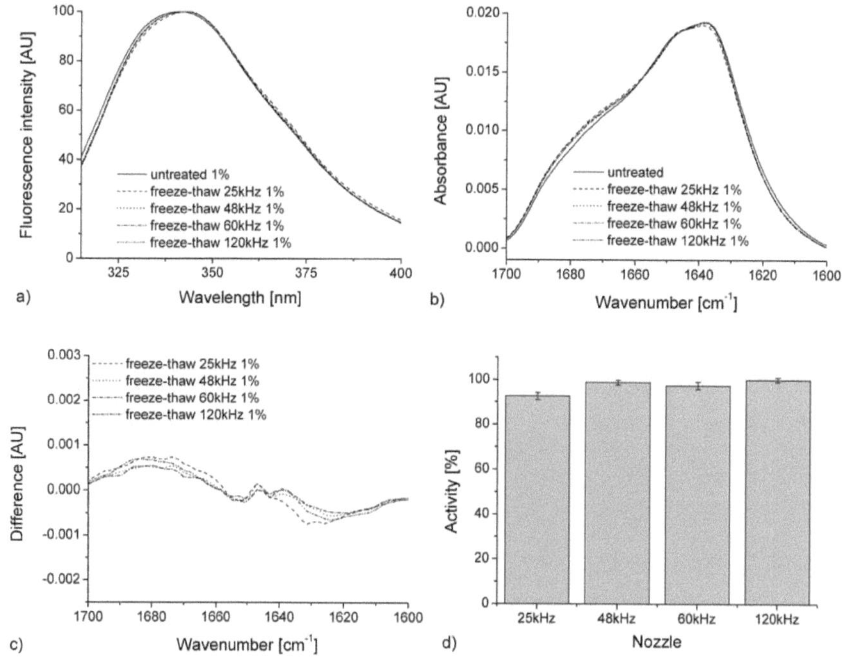

Fig. 6.3: Analysis of 10 mg/mL a-CT freeze-thaw experiments. a) Intrinsic tryptophan fluorescence, b) a-CT amide I bands, c) FTIR difference spectra d) Enzyme activity.

The above displayed reduction in protein damage after quench freezing during SFD has been reported earlier in literature [Sonner et al. 2002; Yu et al. 2006] and is discussed thoroughly in section 6.6 of this thesis.

6.2.3 Spray-freeze-drying experiments

The SFD product was analyzed in the same way as the atomization and freeze-thaw experiments after reconstitution and subsequent centrifugation to eliminate any potential precipitates. In comparison to atomization alone, the removal of water led to further detoriations in protein tertiary structure. Intrinsic tryptophan fluorescence exhibited bathochrome shifts irrespective of the nozzle type used. However, subtle differences caused by the individual nozzles were still present. Damage by the 60 kHz nozzle transposed λ_{max} by only 1.1 nm followed by SFD performed at 120 kHz (+1.3 nm) and 48 kHz (+1.7 nm). Spray-freeze-drying using the 25 kHz nozzle again inflicted the highest detoriations to tertiary structure indicated by a bathochrome shift to 344.4 nm (+2.9 nm) (Fig. 6.4a).

Changes in protein secondary structure also indicated elevated stress levels for a-CT by the removal of water. By comparing the spectra, slight broadening and loss of intensity became apparent for the area-normalized amide I bands. These effects are typical for damage to secondary structure [Costantino et al. 1998], and are observable especially for the 25 kHz SFD product (Fig. 6.4b).

Quantification via calibration curves confirmed the reduction of native structures in favor of aggregated strands for the 25 kHz SFD product (α-helix: -2.9%, intramolecular β-sheet +0.4%, intermolecular β-sheet +2.0%). The other ultrasound nozzles showed similar increases in intermolecular β-sheet, indicating slight aggregation as well (see Table 6.3). However, the decline in α-helix, visible in the amide I band of the 25kHz SFD product, was unique, suggesting that highest protein damage was caused by this nozzle (see Fig. 6.4c).

Compared to the atomization experiments, a-CT enzyme activity was further reduced by the complete SFD cycle (Fig. 6.4c). Results were close for all nozzles examined, providing values between 77% (25 kHz) and 81% (60 kHz) of the activity of the untreated protein. The particles generated by the 25 kHz nozzle showed overall highest loss in stability, indicating that damage inflicted during atomization was present in the final product as well.

Table 6.3: Changes to a-CT secondary structure after the complete SFD process performed at low concentrations.

Nozzle type	α-Helix	Intramol. β-sheet	Intermol. β-sheet
25 kHz nozzle	-2.9%	+0.4%	+2.0%
48 kHz nozzle	-1.0%	-0.3%	+1.7%
60 kHz nozzle	-0.3%	±0.0%	+1.3%
120 kHz nozzle	±0.0%	-0.9%	+1.5%

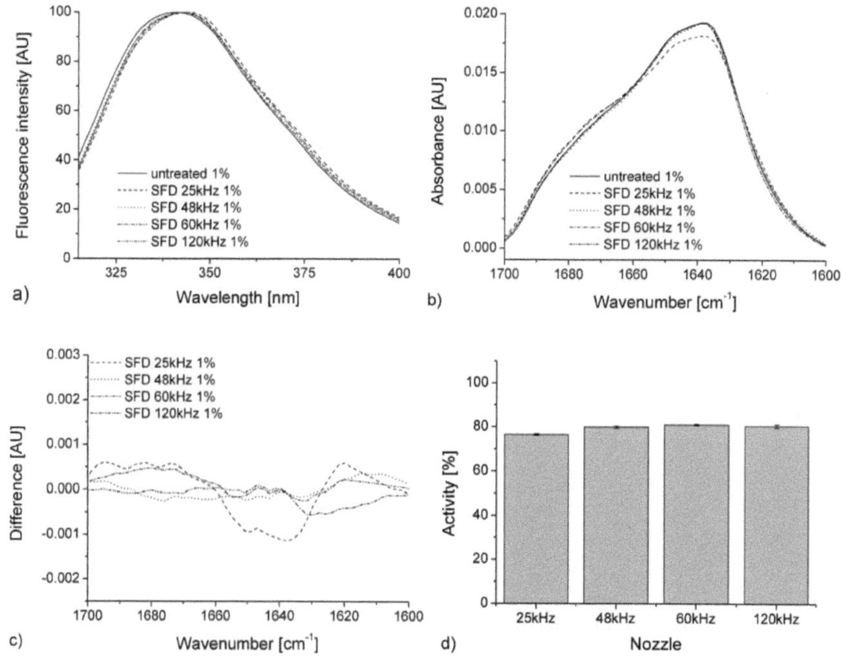

Fig. 6.4: Stability evaluation of the 10 mg/mL a-CT SFD experiments. a) Fluorescence spectra, b) FTIR amide I bands, c) Difference spectra calculated by subtracting the SFD amide I bands from the untreated sample, d) Enzyme activity assay.

SEM pictures of the individual a-CT SFD products with low protein concentrations are displayed in Fig. 6.5a-d. The sponge-like appearance in combination with a very high porosity are typical for particles generated by spray-freeze-drying [Costantino et al. 2002]. Due to the very rapid freezing rate of the droplet spray in liquid nitrogen, very fine ice particles are formed [Hottot et al. 2007]. This led to a highly porous structure during water removal and as consequence to a huge specific surface area. The samples also exhibited drastic reduction in bulk density compared to the lyophilized protein delivered by the manufacturer. Due to the low initial solid content, the spherical shape of the frozen droplets could not be retained in the SFD particles [Sonner 2002]. Therefore, the final product resembled more lyophilized cakes manufactured by conventional freeze-drying rather than distinct particles.

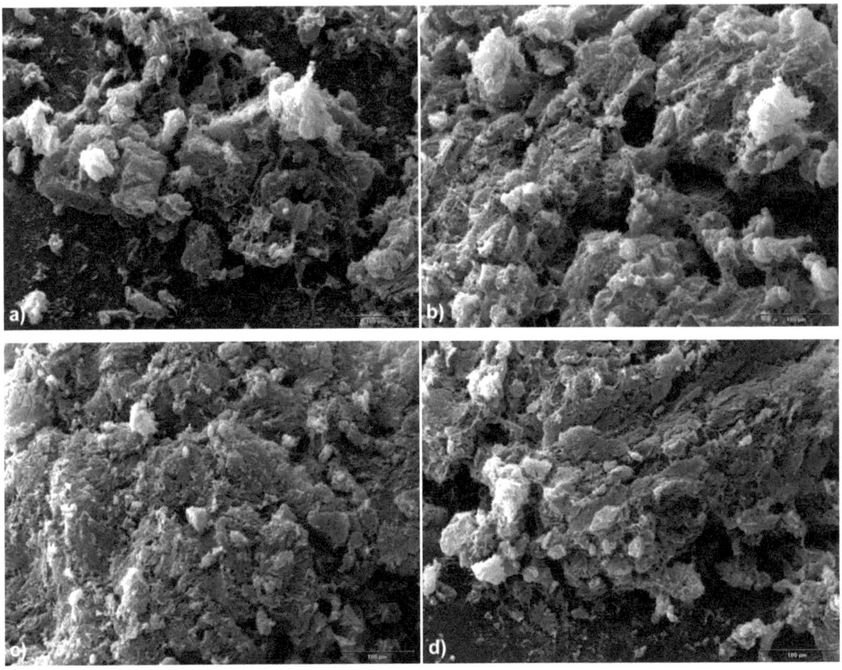

Fig. 6.5: SEM pictures of a-CT particles after SFD of 10 mg/mL solutions using different ultrasonic nozzles: a) 25 kHz, b) 48 kHz, c) 60 kHz, and d) 120 kHz (all 250x magnification).

6.3 Human serum albumin particles from low concentrated solutions (10 mg/mL)

6.3.1 Atomization experiments

HSA tertiary and secondary structure, when analyzed from redissolved samples, has previously shown a high degree of stability during lyophilization [Lin et al. 2000]. Hence, it should be interesting to see if its native conformations would still be preserved during the additional stress posed during SFD. HSA contains one tryptophan residue (Trp 214) [Muzammil et al. 1999] which exhibited a fluorescence maximum at 348.7 nm (sdv=0.03 nm) after dissolution in water at a concentration of 10 mg/mL. As λ_{max} of free tryptophan in aqueous solution is located at 353 nm [Zhou et al. 1997], it seems that the amino acid was already positioned in a rather hydrophilic environment at the outside of the protein. During the atomization step HSA exhibited excellent stability irrespective of the nozzle type used. Fluorescence maxima of the low concentrated solution underwent only subtle shifts to higher wavelengths between 349.0 nm (sdv=0.14 nm) at 48 kHz and 349.4 nm (sdv=0.48 nm) at 60 kHz, indicating no changes in protein tertiary structure (Fig. 6.6a).

Native secondary structure of HSA consisted of 78.8% α-helix, 10.2% intramolecular β-sheet and only 0.9% intermolecular β-sheet. During the spraying step, helical content dropped by maximal 2.8% while intra- and intermolecular β-sheet increased by 1.6% and 0.7%, respectively (Table 6.4). These changes were still within the boundaries of error defined in chapter 5.4.1. Therefore, the alterations to secondary structure were considered negligible, regardless of the nozzle type installed (Fig. 6.6b).

Table 6.4: Effect of atomization on HSA secondary structure (10 mg/mL).

Nozzle type	α-Helix	Intramol. β-sheet	Intermol. β-sheet
25 kHz nozzle	-2.1%	+1.4%	+0.2%
48 kHz nozzle	-2.7%	+1.0%	+0.7%
60 kHz nozzle	-2.5%	+1.6%	+0.4%
120 kHz nozzle	-1.6%	+1.0%	+0.5%
Two-fluid nozzle	-2.8%	+1.5%	+0.3%

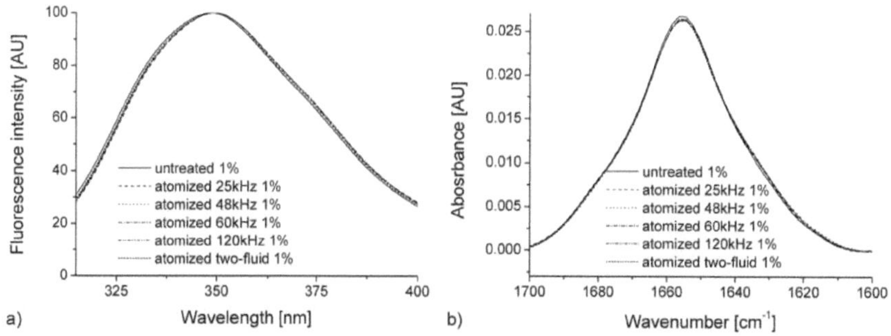

Fig. 6.6: Stability of HSA concerning atomization experiments. a) Fluorescence and b) FTIR spectra indicated no changes in protein tertiary or secondary structure.

For HSA, the atomization step at low concentrations seemed to be rather unproblematic regarding protein tertiary and secondary structure. In contrast to a-CT, even the 25 kHz nozzle was not able to induce noticeable damage.

6.3.2 Freeze-thaw experiments

Quench freezing and subsequent thawing at room temperature of the 10 mg/mL HSA solution had only little effect on its tertiary and secondary structure. In fluorescence spectroscopy, the subtle redshift of λ_{max} between 0.3 nm (25 kHz) and 0.7 nm (48 kHz) did not indicate a reorientation of the tryptophan amino acid after freezing and thawing (Fig. 6.7a). In comparison to atomization alone, HSA fluorescence maxima underwent wavelength shifts of similar dimensions after the freeze-thawing step.

Protein secondary structure, however, experienced minor, but still noticeable changes (Fig. 6.7b). α-helix dropped by values between 3.0% (120 kHz) and 5.7% (48 kHz) while intramolecular β-sheet rose by values between 1.4% and 3.0% respectively (Table 6.5). Interestingly, the intermolecular β-sheet content did not change substantially and increased only by 0.8% at the most (48 kHz).

As with the 10 mg/mL a-CT experiments, it seems that part of the helical HSA secondary structure was reorganized in intramolecular β-sheet during quench freezing. This re-arrangement, however, did not lead to the formation of aggregates as neither substantial shifts of λ_{max} nor increases in intermolecular β-sheet were detectable. Therefore, it seems that rapid freezing slightly favored the creation of β-sheet conformations for both proteins.

Table 6.5: Changes to HSA secondary structure after the freeze-thaw experiments (10 mg/mL).

Nozzle type	α-Helix	Intramol. β-sheet	Intermol. β-sheet
25 kHz nozzle	-4.6%	+2.5%	+0.5%
48 kHz nozzle	-5.7%	+3.0%	+0.8%
60 kHz nozzle	-3.5%	+1.4%	+0.8%
120 kHz nozzle	-3.0%	+1.6%	+0.5%

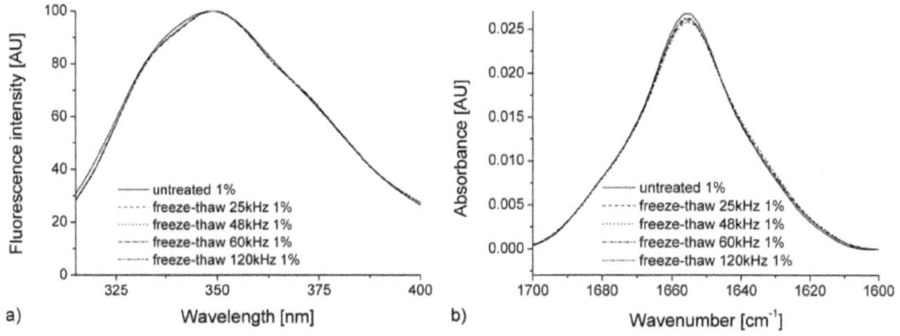

Fig. 6.7: a) Fluorescence and b) FTIR amide I spectra after freezing and subsequent thawing of 10 mg/mL HSA solutions.

6.3.3 Spray-freeze-drying experiments

Subjecting the 10 mg/mL HSA solutions to the complete SFD process didn't have noticeable effects on protein stability either. Minor redshifts were detectable by fluorescence spectroscopy, resulting in λ_{max} values between 349.1 nm (48 kHz) and 349.4 nm (25 kHz) equivalent to a maximum increase by 0.7 nm (Fig. 6.8a). The extent of protein damage was comparable to the one detected during the atomization and freeze-thaw experiments. Hence, neither atomizing nor freezing nor water removal seemed to have noticeable detrimental effects on HSA tertiary structure.

Changes to secondary structure were once again mostly within the margin of error. Results of the 25 kHz nozzle showed highest transitions from α-helix to intra- and intermolecular β-sheets. Helical contents dropped by 3.2% while β-sheets rose by 2.5% and 0.8%, respectively (Fig. 6.8b). This means that slightly elevated processing stress could be detected after the complete SFD process if the 25 kHz nozzle design was applied for atomization. However, the observed changes were still too small to be considered substantial at the investigated concentration (Table 6.6). The other nozzles caused even less alterations to native conformations. In comparison to a-CT, damage to secondary structure was of lower extent, indicating superior HSA stability during the treatment steps.

In summary, HSA proofed to be a very stable protein during spray-freeze-drying. Neither secondary nor tertiary structure was damaged extensively during any of the steps analyzed. Therefore, SFD of low concentrated HSA solutions using ultrasound nozzles showed excellent overall protein stability.

Table 6.6: The effect of the complete spray-freeze-drying process on HSA secondary structure (c=10 mg/mL).

Nozzle type	α-Helix	Intramol. β-sheet	Intermol. β-sheet
25 kHz nozzle	-3.2%	+2.5%	+0.8%
48 kHz nozzle	-0.5%	+0.6%	+0.2%
60 kHz nozzle	-0.7%	+0.1%	+0.4%
120 kHz nozzle	+2.1%	+0.2%	+0.3%

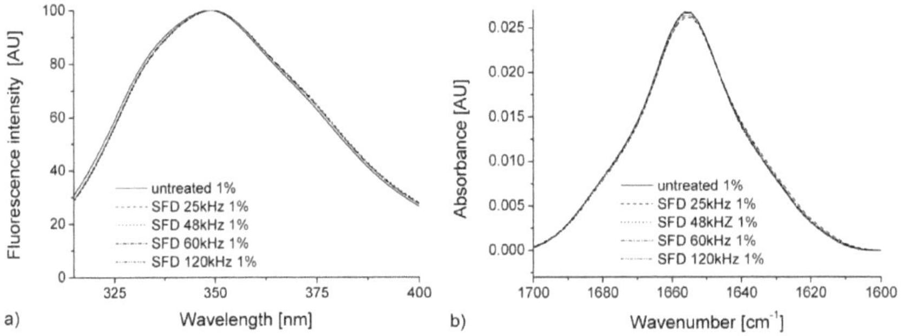

Fig. 6.8: Effect of SFD experiments performed with different ultrasound nozzles on the a) tertiary structure and b) secondary structure of HSA.

As can be seen in Fig. 6.9, no spherical particles could be formed by SFD using the low concentrated HSA solutions. These results, in conjunction with the ones obtained for low concentrated a-CT solutions, supported the findings by Sonner [2002] that a minimum solid content is essential to form spherical particles during SFD. In addition, the choice of nozzle seemed to have no influence on the macroscopic appearance of the SFD product of low concentrated HSA solutions, always resulting in highly porous and sponge-like particles.

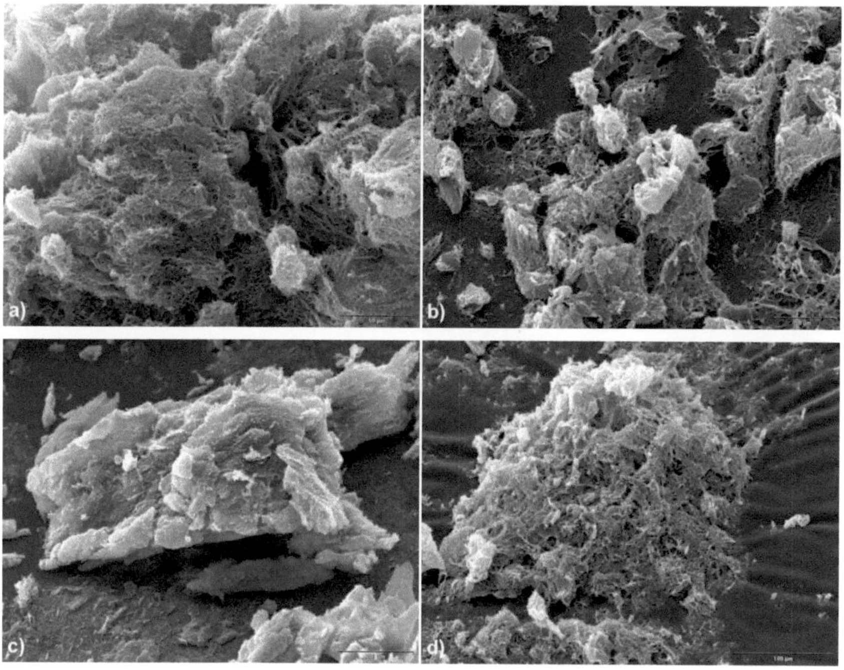

Fig. 6.9: SEM pictures of 10 mg/mL SFD HSA solutions showing structures comparable to the 10 mg/mL a-CT particles: a) 25 kHz (500x), b) 48 kHz (500x), c) 60 kHz (300x) and d) 120 kHz (400x).

6.4 α-Chymotrypsin particles from high concentrated solutions (100 mg/mL)

6.4.1 Atomization experiments

Increasing the solid content to 100 mg/mL had noticeable effects on the untreated a-CT solution even though samples were diluted before analysis (see chapters 4.5 and 4.6) Secondary structure showed a slight decrease in native conformations as the α-helix content dropped by 0.8% to 14.2%, while intermolecular β-sheet increased by 0.5% to 5.8%. These changes were accompanied by a wavelength shift of λ_{max} from 341.5 nm to 342.4 nm detected by fluorescence spectroscopy. While differences in secondary structure alone could still be caused by artifacts measured at low concentrations, the simultaneous alteration in fluorescence maximum strongly suggested concentration-dependent changes in protein structure.

The amount of damage inflicted to the enzyme during atomization was dependent on the nozzle type used. The 60 kHz nozzle exhibited lowest detoriations to tertiary structure, only shifting the fluorescence maximum by 0.6 nm to 343.0 nm. Two-fluid, 48 kHz and 120 kHz nozzles inflicted comparable protein stress (λ_{max} lay between 343.7 nm and 344.9 nm) which corresponds to moderate disorganizations of tertiary structure. However, atomization at 25 kHz led to obvious damage. λ_{max} shifted to 349.7 nm – a wavelength near to the fluorescence maximum of free tryptophan. This indicated that the tryptophan residues that are normally located inside the protein were moved to the periphery as tertiary structure was severely altered (Fig. 6.10a).

Analysis by FTIR spectroscopy indicated that changes to secondary and tertiary structures occurred simultaneously. Atomization by two-fluid, 60 kHz and 120 kHz nozzles inflicted the lowest damage, increasing the amount of intermolecular β-sheet by 0.3% – 0.6%. The 48 kHz nozzle exhibited stronger protein stress (intermolecular β-sheet +1.2%), while the 25 kHz nozzle showed highest detrimental effects (see Table 6.7). Native structure was reduced by 3.3% (α-helix) and 2.8% (intramolecular β-sheet), respectively, while intermolecular β-sheets increased by 5.1% (Fig. 6.10b) which corresponded to noticeable aggregate formation. By subtracting the spectrum of the untreated protein from the atomized solutions, differences become even more prominent (Fig. 6.10c) indicating massive damage by the 25 kHz nozzle.

a-CT activity assay also indicated different stress levels by the individual nozzle designs. The 60 kHz nozzle only showed little effect on overall enzyme stability, retrieving a residual activity of 95.3%. Atomization by two-fluid, 48 kHz and 120 kHz nozzles noticeably affected protein stability by reducing its activity to values between 82.0% and 88.3%. Once more, a-CT suffered strongest damage by the 25 kHz nozzle resulting in a residual activity of only 63.7% (Fig. 6.10d). In addition, protein damage at 25 kHz was macroscopically observable, as the atomized solution showed noticeable precipitation and foaming.

It is important to note that results for the 25 kHz nozzle showed noticeable variability not only in the enzyme activity assay (see sdv in Fig. 6.10d), but also in the FTIR and fluorescence spectra. The same was true for the 120 kHz nozzle, but to a lower extent. A thorough discussion of possible reasons can be found in chapters 7.4.5 and 8.2.4.

Table 6.7: Influence of atomization conditions on the secondary structure of high concentrated a-CT solutions.

Nozzle type	α-Helix	Intramol. β-sheet	Intermol. β-sheet
25 kHz nozzle	-3.3%	-2.8%	+5.1%
48 kHz nozzle	-0.3%	-1.4%	+1.2%
60 kHz nozzle	-0.1%	-0.9%	+0.5%
120 kHz nozzle	-0.2%	-0.5%	+0.3%
Two-fluid nozzle	+0.3%	-1.0%	+0.6%

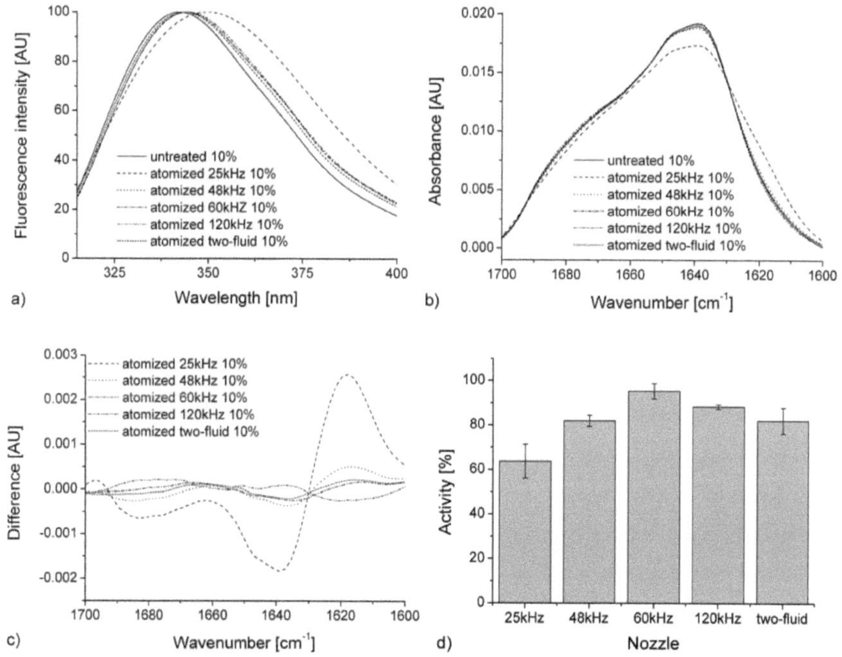

Fig. 6.10: Stability of a-CT at a concentration of 100 mg/mL during the atomization experiments. a) Fluorescence spectra, b) FTIR amide I bands, c) Difference spectra of the FTIR amide I bands, d) UV activity assay.

6.4.2 Freeze-thaw experiments

Quench-freezing of the chymotrypsin droplet spray could preserve protein stability to a certain extent. In concurrence to the findings presented in chapter 6.2.2, the enzyme suffered lower damage than during atomization alone.

Compared to the spraying procedure, the fluorescence maximum showed a hypsochrome shift most prominent for the 25 kHz nozzle from 349.7 nm (atomized) back to 344.5 nm (freeze-thaw). The other nozzles even exhibited tertiary structures close to the untreated protein, resulting in λ_{max} values between 342.5 nm (120 kHz) and 342.9 nm (48 kHz) (Fig. 6.11a). Hence, a-CT tertiary structure proved to be more stable if the droplets were instantly frozen after the spraying step.

Damage to secondary structure was also mostly averted by freezing in LN_2. The considerable increase in intermolecular β-sheet during atomization at 25 kHz (+5.1%) was reduced, resulting in an increase by only 1.6% compared to the untreated protein. For the other nozzles a slight reduction in intermolecular β-sheet by 0.3%-0.4% was even detectable (again in comparison to the native conformation) (Fig. 6.11b). The decrease in intermolecular β-sheet was linked to minor increases in intramolecular β-sheet which rose by values between 0.2% (48 kHz) and 0.9% (120 kHz) (Table 6.8). These changes can easily be observed by comparing the difference spectra of the freeze-thaw experiments with the ones from atomization alone (Fig. 6.11c). It seemed that the rapid freezing rates favored the generation of intramolecular β-sheet at both high and low concentrations. However, the changes were rather subtle and near the limits of detection which makes definite conclusion difficult.

The enzyme activity assay confirmed the results detected by FTIR and fluorescence spectroscopy. The most obvious changes were visible for the 25 kHz nozzle which could retain 80.5% of its activity. This equals an increase by 16.8% compared to the atomization experiments. For the other nozzles examined, enzyme activity was either very close to (e.g. 60 kHz, 120 kHz) or even above the values (48 kHz) determined during spraying (Fig. 6.11d). In case of the 60 kHz and 120 kHz nozzles, any further stabilization was obviously very hard to accomplish as the residual activity was still very high after the atomization step.

Table 6.8: Changes to a-CT secondary structure due to quench freezing (100 mg/mL).

Nozzle type	α-Helix	Intramol. β-sheet	Intermol. β-sheet
25 kHz nozzle	-2.0%	+0.6%	+1.6%
48 kHz nozzle	±0.0%	+0.2%	-0.3%
60 kHz nozzle	-0.2%	+0.6%	-0.3%
120 kHz nozzle	-0.4%	+0.9%	-0.4%

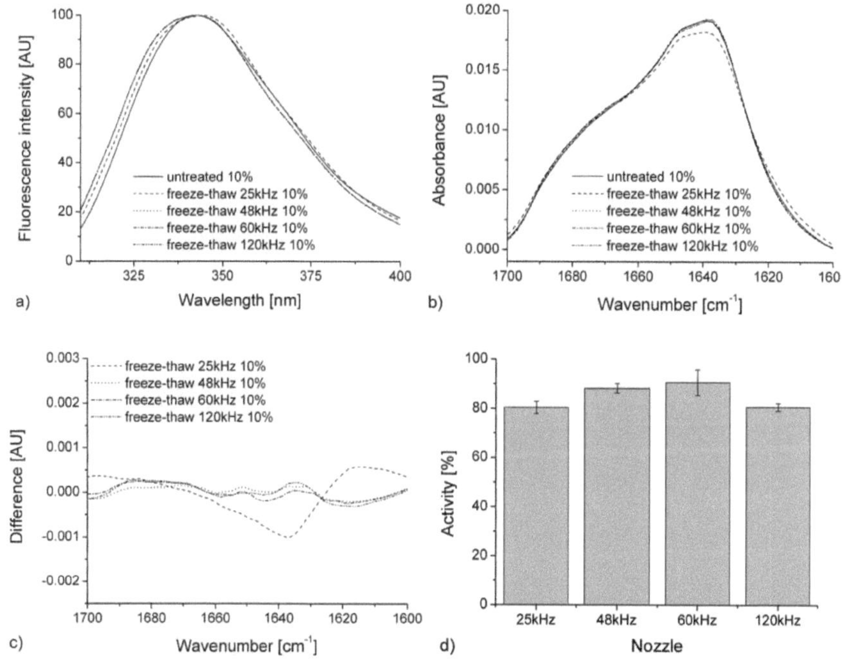

Fig. 6.11: Damage to a-CT due to freezing and subsequent thawing at high concentrations. a) Fluorescence spectra, b) FTIR amide I bands, c) FTIR difference spectra, generated by subtracting the untreated from processed amide I bands, d) UV activity assay.

6.4.3 Spray-freeze-drying experiments

After having performed the complete SFD cycle with different nozzle types, discrepancies between the 100 mg/mL a-CT products became even more evident. During reconstitution, a large fraction of the particles atomized at 25 kHz could not be redissolved, leading to insoluble aggregates that had to be removed by centrifugation. Spraying with the other ultrasonic nozzles, however, inflicted little or no macroscopic observable insoluble aggregates in the final particles.

Best results regarding a-CT stability were accomplished after the SFD process using the 60 kHz nozzle. The reconstituted particles showed a slight wavelength shift by 1.7 nm to 344.2 nm (Fig. 6.12a). The 48 kHz and 120 kHz nozzles inflicted the same levels of damage to protein tertiary structure: λ_{max} was transposed by 4.2 nm and 3.6 nm at 48 kHz and 120 kHz, respectively. By comparing those redshifts with the ones from the atomization experiments, further damage during the freeze-drying step became obvious. However, results for the 25 kHz nozzle were surprisingly good. The corresponding λ_{max} at 345.0 nm suggested even less detoriations to tertiary structure than at 48 kHz and 120 kHz which is unlikely considering the results of atomization experiments.

The changes in a-CT secondary structure were associated with the changes in its tertiary structure (Table 6.9). Intermolecular β-sheet rose slightly by 0.7% after SFD employing the 60 kHz nozzle. Spray-freeze-drying with the 48 kHz and 120 kHz nozzles increased aggregation of a-CT substantially, increasing intermolecular β-sheet contents by 4.2% and 3.5% respectively (Fig. 6.12b). This indicates higher damage than during atomization alone, and thus changes should have been caused by the removal of water. As for fluorescence spectroscopy, evaluation of a-CT secondary structure after the 25 kHz SFD experiment surprisingly suggested increased protein stability over the 48 kHz and 120 kHz nozzles, showing an increase in intermolecular β-sheet by only 2.5% (Fig. 6.12c).

The relatively good results of the 25 kHz nozzle had to be revised after evaluation of the enzyme activity assay. Overall a-CT stability of the reconstituted particles was reduced to 47.1% (Fig. 6.12d) indicating that the protein had suffered severe damage. The most plausible reason for this result is that the fraction of a-CT forming the insoluble aggregates was eliminated by centrifugation, thus lowering the concentration of the sample. Fluorescence emission was only evaluated for the position of the intensity normalized λ_{max}. Therefore, only the relatively undamaged fractions were analyzed, leading to false positive results. Changes in concentration could not be distinguished by this method of analysis. FTIR spectroscopy suffered from similar problems because the amide I band was area normalized before quantification. Enzyme activity, however, is strongly dependent on the concentration of the reconstituted solution, making the differences obvious. Damage to overall stability by the remaining nozzles was in concurrence with the results determined for secondary and tertiary structures. Lowest detrimental effects were achieved for the SFD cycle at 60 kHz, leading to a residual activity of 82.3% while the 48 kHz and 120 kHz experiments showed activity values of 74.0% and 74.7% respectively.

As observed in chapter 6.4.1, results of the 25 kHz nozzle showed again noticeable variations. Reduced reproducibility was also observed for the 120 kHz and 48 kHz nozzle, but to a far lower extent.

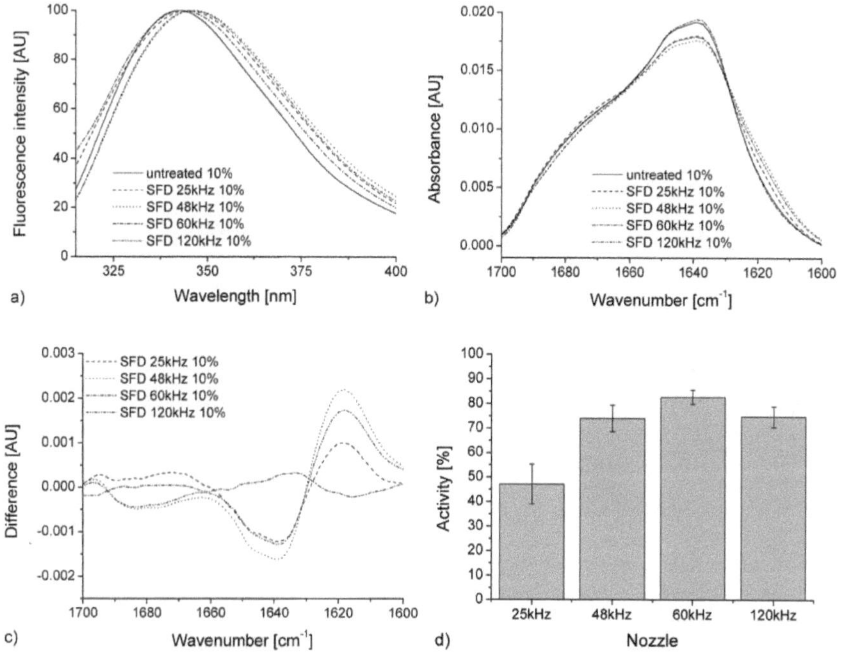

Fig. 6.12: Damage to a-CT after the complete SFD process performed at a concentration of 100 mg/mL. a) Fluorescence spectra, b) FTIR amide I bands, c) Difference spectra calculated by subtracting the untreated from the processed amide I bands, d) UV activity assay.

Table 6.9: Changes to a-CT secondary structure due to spray-freeze-drying (100 mg/mL).

Nozzle type	α-Helix	Intramol. β-sheet	Intermol. β-sheet
25 kHz nozzle	-2.0%	-0.5%	+2.5%
48 kHz nozzle	-3.2%	-2.9%	+4.2%
60 kHz nozzle	-0.6%	+0.6%	+0.7%
120 kHz nozzle	-2.1%	-2.2%	+3.5%

The pure a-CT particles generated by SFD are presented in Fig. 6.13a-d. SEM pictures revealed a spherical shape with highly porous surfaces. These findings are typical for SFD products manufactured from intermediate concentrated solutions and have been discussed earlier in the literature [Sonner et al. 2002; Wang et al. 2004; van Drooge et al. 2005]. Increasing nozzle frequencies led to decreasing particle sizes, indicating that the shape and size of the droplets has been preserved throughout the lyophilization process.

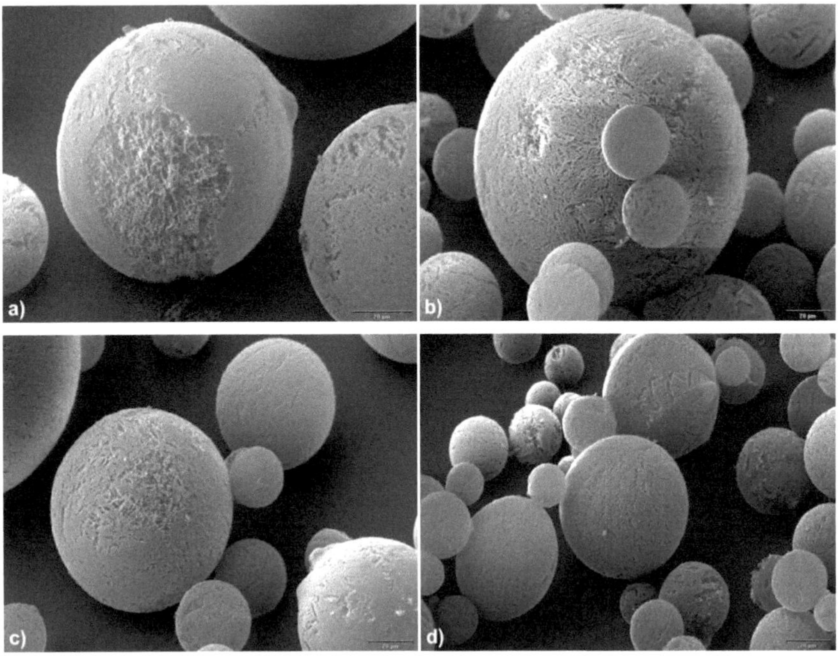

Fig. 6.13: SEM pictures of pure a-CT particles generated from 100 mg/mL solutions. a) 25 kHz (240x), b) 48 kHz (750x), c) 60 kHz (750x), d) 120 kHz (750x).

6.5 Human serum albumin particles from high concentrated solutions (100 mg/mL)

6.5.1 Atomization experiments

By increasing the protein concentration to 100 mg/mL, slight changes to the tertiary and secondary structure of untreated HSA were detectable even though samples were diluted before analysis (see sections 4.5.2 and 4.6). The fluorescence maximum of the untreated solution shifted from 348.7 nm to 349.5 nm, while secondary structure underwent minor changes as well: α-helix dropped from 78.8% to 77.6%, whereas intra- and intermolecular β-sheet increased from 10.2% to 10.8% and from 0.9% to 1.0%, respectively. This is in agreement with the observations made for the a-CT solutions in section 6.4.1.

No substantial differences in protein fluorescence maxima could be observed after the atomization step (Fig. 6.14a). Redshifts lay between 0.2 nm (48 kHz) and 0.7 nm (120 kHz), which corresponds to the bathochrome shifts determined for 10 mg/mL solutions. Therefore, HSA tertiary structure exhibited similar high levels of stability during atomization at low and high concentrations.

Damage to HSA secondary structure was also in a close range for all nozzle types examined (Fig. 6.14b). Helical content dropped by values between 1.1% (48 kHz) and 2.0% (120 kHz) while intra- and intermolecular β-sheet rose by 1.0% and 0.4% at most (see Table 6.10).

Table 6.10: Effects of atomization conditions on high concentrated HSA solutions.

Nozzle type	α-Helix	Intramol. β-sheet	Intermol. β-sheet
25 kHz nozzle	-1.6%	+1.0%	+0.4%
48 kHz nozzle	-1.1%	+0.6%	+0.3%
60 kHz nozzle	-1.8%	+1.0%	+0.2%
120 kHz nozzle	-2.0%	+0.9%	+0.2%
Two-fluid nozzle	-1.5%	+0.6%	+0.3%

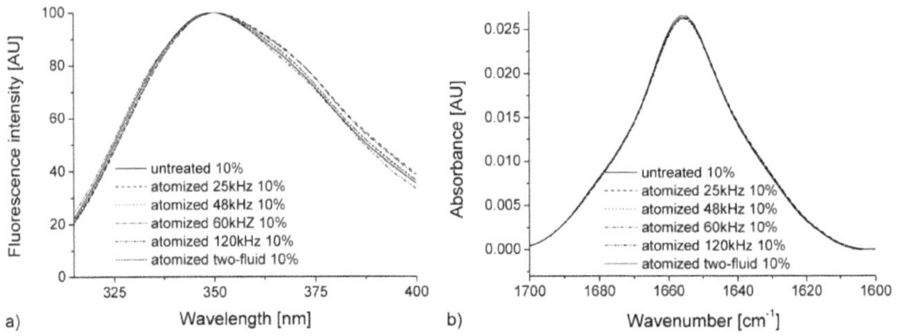

Fig. 6.14: Changes to a) protein tertiary and b) secondary structure of 100 mg/mL HSA solutions due to atomization by different nozzle designs.

These minor changes to native conformations were within the limit of detection and should therefore be regarded with caution. The 25 kHz nozzle was not able to induce higher levels of damage than the other nozzles which was surprising considering the 100 mg/mL a-CT atomization experiments.

Regarding protein secondary and tertiary structure, HSA proved to be very stable during atomization if ultrasonic nozzles were applied. The same was true for two-fluid nozzles if a rather large droplet size – and thereby a small specific surface area – were produced.

6.5.2 Freeze-thaw experiments

Analysis of the 100 mg/mL samples after freezing and subsequent thawing exhibited marginal changes in protein tertiary structure. The fluorescence spectrum of HSA, generated by its only tryptophan residue, showed a slight blueshift of the whole band in comparison to the untreated protein (Fig. 6.15a). Fluorescence maxima, on the other hand, almost stayed at the same wavelength as the native sample. This could indicate subtle changes in protein tertiary structure as the shape of the fluorescence band is known to be defined by different underlying tryptophan peaks (similar to the composition of the amide I band) [Kumar et al. 2005]. However, those findings were not included in the evaluation as λ_{max} was considered the most straight-forward approach for determining changes in tertiary structure.

The 60 kHz freeze-thawed sample experienced the highest hypsochrome shift to 348.5 nm (untreated: 349.5 nm). Hence, it seems that the microenvironment of tryptophan has been changed towards a more defined state in an overall slightly less hydrophilic location without affecting λ_{max} much. This effect was also detected for the other protein samples analyzed, but to a lesser extent (see sections 6.2.2, 6.3.2 and 6.4.2). In those cases, λ_{max} was shifted hypsochrome in comparison to atomization alone but never beyond the signal of the native protein.

Secondary structure also underwent noticeable changes compared to the untreated protein: α-helix was reduced by up to 3.6% after quench freezing, whereas intra- and intermolecular β-sheet rose by maximal 2.1% and 0.6%, respectively (Fig. 6.15b). Surprisingly, the 25 kHz nozzle induced roughly the same level of refolding as the 48 kHz design. Alterations caused by the two higher frequency nozzles only lay within the margin of error and were not considered significant (see Table 6.11). Hence, HSA exhibited a behavior similar to previously examined secondary structures after freeze-thawing: Loss in native α-helix led to an increase in intramolecular β-sheet. The formation of aggregates could not be ascertained as intermolecular β-sheet only increased by a small amount.

In summary, no elevated damage was observable for the high concentrated HSA samples after flash freezing in LN_2 and subsequent thawing. The slight changes in tertiary and secondary structure do not seem to be linked to aggregation but rather to a minor protein refolding.

Table 6.11: The influence of freeze-thaw experiments on the secondary structure of high concentrated a-CT solutions.

Nozzle type	α-Helix	Intramol. β-sheet	Intermol. β-sheet
25 kHz nozzle	-3.4%	+1.9%	+0.6%
48 kHz nozzle	-3.6%	+2.1%	+0.6%
60 kHz nozzle	-2.2%	+1.5%	+0.3%
120 kHz nozzle	-1.0%	+0.9%	+0.2%

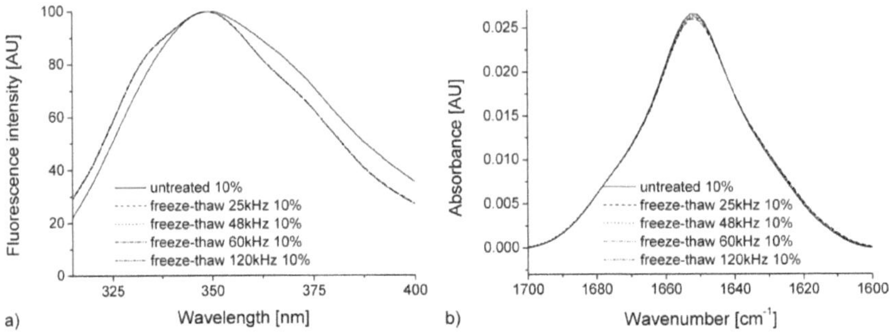

Fig. 6.15: a) Fluorescence and b) FTIR spectra of a 100 mg/mL HSA solution after freezing and subsequent thawing at room temperature. Fluorescence spectra match very closely and therefore appear as only one graph in the above diagram.

6.5.3 Spray-freeze-drying experiments

Finally, stability of HSA after the complete SFD process was evaluated. Wavelengths of the fluorescence maxima underwent minor changes, increasing by 0.5 nm-1.0 nm (Fig. 6.16a) which is comparable to the effect of atomization alone. Only the overall appearance of the 25 kHz spectrum indicated further differences to the untreated protein. The shape of the fluorescence band exhibited a new shoulder at 330 nm while λ_{max} was shifted to 350.5 nm, indicating subtle damage to native conformations. For the other nozzle frequencies examined, HSA tertiary structure remained mostly unaltered during the complete SFD process.

Results from FTIR analysis, on the other hand, suggest that HSA stability was slightly affected during SFD (Fig. 6.16b). Helical content dropped by 4.6% at most using the 25 kHz nozzle for spraying, while the remaining nozzles exhibited a reduction in α-helix content between 3.3% and 1.6% (see Table 6.12). β-sheets showed little changes as well, with the 25 kHz nozzle inflicting the highest damage (intramolecular β-sheet +2.6%, intermolecular β-sheet +0.8%). In contrast to a-CT, damage to native structure was independent of the concentration used as both 10 and 100 mg/mL solutions showed similar effects.

In summary, overall stability of HSA secondary and tertiary structure proved to be relatively high during SFD for all nozzles and processing conditions examined. Only the 25 kHz design showed slight differences in comparison to the other nozzles. However, differences were marginal and nowhere near the extent observed in the a-CT experiments. Increasing the concentration of HSA did not lead to a higher structural susceptibility in regard to the individual processing steps.

Table 6.12: Quantification of changes to HSA secondary structure after spray-freeze-drying from high concentrated solutions.

Nozzle type	α-Helix	Intramol. β-sheet	Intermol. β-sheet
25 kHz nozzle	-4.6%	+2.6%	+0.8%
48 kHz nozzle	-3.3%	+1.7%	+0.5%
60 kHz nozzle	-3.5%	+2.1%	+0.3%
120 kHz nozzle	-1.6%	+0.6%	+0.3%

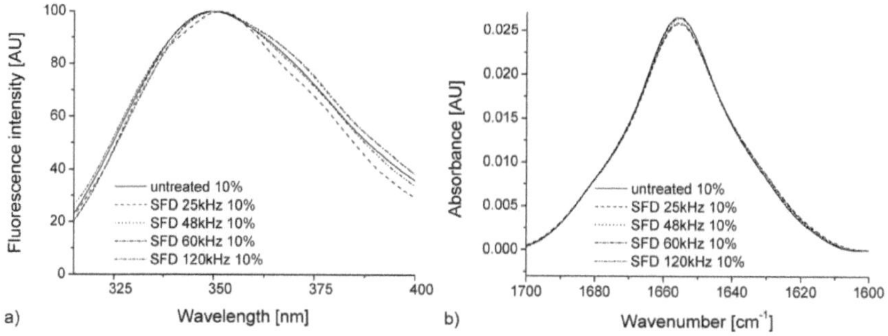

Fig. 6.16: a) Fluorescence and b) FTIR spectroscopy of HSA after the complete SFD process.

As seen with the high concentrated a-CT experiments, 100 mg/mL HSA solutions led to distinct spherical particles (Fig. 6.17a-d). The surface was again highly porous which becomes prominent on Fig. 6.17a where obvious holes are detectable on the larger particles. Otherwise, no differences between SFD particles generated from 100 mg/mL a-CT or HSA solutions were detectable.

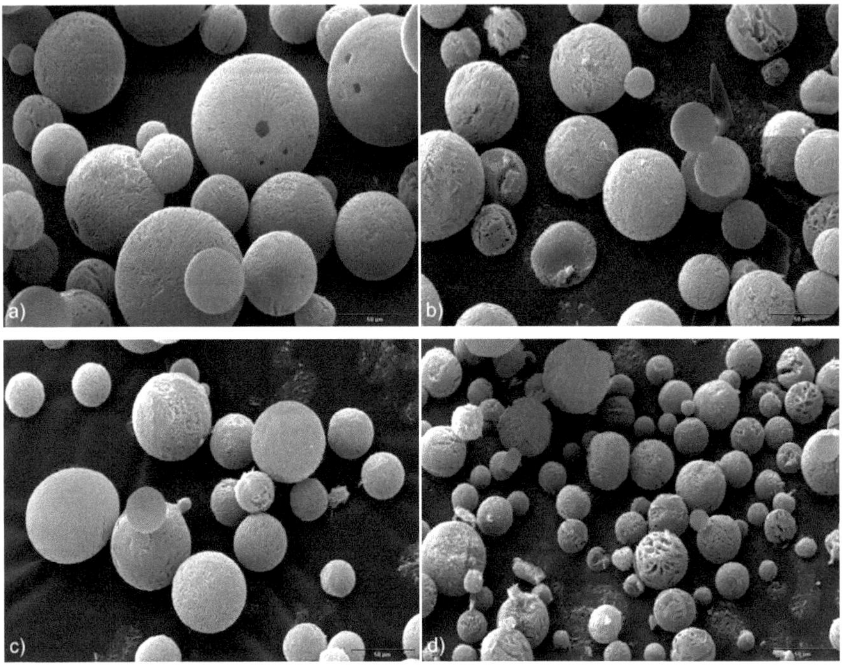

Fig. 6.17: SEM photographs of pure HSA protein particles generated from 100 mg/mL solutions. Each picture was taken at 500x enlargement: a) 25 kHz, b) 48 kHz, c) 60 kHz, d) 120 kHz.

6.6 Overall comparison and discussion

Atomization presents the first critical processing step during SFD [Webb et al. 2002]. Proteins tend to adsorb to the air/liquid interface, and therefore a high specific surface area, e.g. during the spraying step, can favor protein denaturation. This is especially important as different droplet sizes can be produced, depending on the frequency of the ultrasonic nozzle. The smaller the droplets are, the larger the resulting specific surface area becomes. The stability of BSA (which shares a 73% structural similarity with HSA [Gelamo et al. 2000]) during SFD was previously analyzed by Costantino et al. [2000] using a two-fluid nozzle at a wide variety of liquid feed rates and atomizing air-flows. They could correlate an increasing loss of protein monomer with decreasing SFD particle size and increasing powder surface area, especially for a $d_{v,50}$ of 5μm or less. In another study, Yu et al. [2006] discovered that lysozyme particles produced by SFL (see chapter 2.1.2) showed nearly no loss in monomer content or native secondary structure in contrast to the SFD process. Therefore, it was stated that protein damage was predominantly inflicted by its adsorption to the air-liquid interface during the spraying step. Finally, Maa et al. [2000] found out that aggregation during the atomization step seems to be strongly dependent on the protein used. rhDNase and rhMAb were very stable at the air-liquid interface, suggesting that aggregation occurred mainly during the fast freezing or the subsequent drying step. In this thesis, the effect of atomization conditions was dependent on the investigated protein as well. HSA was very stable throughout this processing step irrespective of the concentration or nozzle used. This is surprising at first, considering the damage to BSA detected by Costantino et al. [2000]. However, some important differences must be taken into account when comparing both studies: HSA still exhibits 27% difference to BSA in primary structure, therefore analogous behavior during atomization is not for sure. Additionally, spraying stress was strongly dependent on the atomization conditions applied by the two-fluid nozzle. Strongest aggregation was detected for droplet sizes <5 µm which is far below the droplet diameters in this study. And finally, the FTIR spectra were taken as KBr pellets from the final product. Findings by Lin et al. [2000] suggested that HSA almost completely refolds during the reconstitution from lyophilized powder. This could explain the superior stability of HSA detected in this work.

Results from a-CT, on the other hand, were strongly dependent on nozzle frequency and concentration. According to the findings of Costantino et al. [2000], the nozzle oscillating at the highest frequency should induce the highest protein damage because droplet size is inversely proportional to the atomization frequency. However, this is not the case as the 25 kHz nozzle inflicted highest protein damage at the chosen settings, but generated the lowest specific surface area (see also chapter 6.4). Hence, it seems obvious that more factors than aggregation at the droplet surface are relevant when ultrasonic nozzles are applied for atomization. Possible differences between the individual frequencies in regard to temperature and cavitation are discussed in chapter 7, while adsorption of a-CT to the air/liquid interface and its stabilization by the addition of polysorbat 80 is analyzed in chapter 8.1.

The next step in the SFD process consisted of quench freezing of the fine droplets by LN_2. For both a-CT and HSA, protein stability was equal or even superior to the results determined during the corresponding atomization experiments. This phenomenon was previously described by Sonner et al. [2002] and Yu et al. [2006] using lysozyme as model enzyme. For explanation, they postulated that partial unfolding is being reversed during quench freezing resulting in increased protein stability. As the degree of protein denaturation in the spraying step is known to be proportional to the time frame it has to reach the surface as well as the overall surface area [Costantino et al. 2000], another way of stabilization is plausible: The fine droplets already start to freeze while falling through the vapor phase and solidify completely upon contact with the cryogen. Protein adsorption to the air/liquid interface is therefore substantial reduced which leads to superior stability [Yu et al. 2006]. The first assumption concurs best with the results presented in this work as evaluations indicated that very rapid freezing had subtle but noticeable effects on protein secondary and tertiary structure: The tryptophan residues were preferential buried in little more hydrophobic environments while intramolecular β-sheet content was slightly increased. It has yet to be evaluated if these alterations also somehow affected protein stability in the subsequent freeze-drying step. Furthermore, changes detected within the fluorescence bands of HSA suggested that not all alterations to protein tertiary structure could be determined by evaluating the wavelength maximum (chapter 6.5.2). However, an in-depth investigation of the effect of freezing and subsequent thawing on protein tertiary structure by fluorescence spectroscopy lies beyond the scope of this thesis but should be considered in future work.

When comparing the final HSA and a-CT particles, it becomes noticeable that the removal of water can impose another stress factor during SFD. For HSA only little effects were visible after reconstitution of the product, while a-CT experienced noticeable reductions in stability. Enzyme activity always was below the values determined for atomization and freeze-thawing, indicating highest damage after the complete process. Yu et al. [2006] analyzed SFD stepwise for a 5 mg/mL lysozyme solution in a way similar to the experiments performed in this thesis. However, evaluation of the complete SFD process yielded slightly elevated lysozyme activity compared to the atomization experiments alone (86.3% vs. 78.3%) which is contrary to the findings in this thesis. This unsuspected result was explained by the fact that the smallest droplets (containing the protein fraction with strongest adsorption to the air/liquid interface) could escape the bowl containing LN_2 due to the strong atomizing air flow of the two-fluid nozzle. In consequence, the enzyme activity assay yielded false positive results. The explanation seems plausible as the SFD experiments in this thesis were mostly conducted using ultrasonic nozzles. They generated a "soft spray" that was not propelled by airflow and therefore the percentage of small droplets that were able to reach the surface of LN_2 should have increased noticeably.

Alterations in secondary and tertiary structure of the 100 mg/mL a-CT solution appeared to be connected to changes in its residual enzyme activity. Therefore, investigation of a linear relationship between the different methods of analysis seemed promising. Experiments from the 25 kHz SFD experiments were excluded as results from FTIR and fluorescence spectroscopy were considered as outliers (see section 6.4.3). For FTIR, a moderate correlation could be achieved by plotting the changes of intermolecular β-sheet (Fig. 6.18a) against a-CT activity, giving a R^2 value of 0.715 while the relationship between shifts in fluorescence maxima and enzyme activity resulted in a R^2 value of 0.706 (Fig. 6.18b). A stronger correlation would have been surprising as these methods of analysis focus on very different aspects of the enzyme. Still, the results follow the same trend and thus support the analytical approach performed in this thesis for evaluating protein stability during spray-freeze-drying.

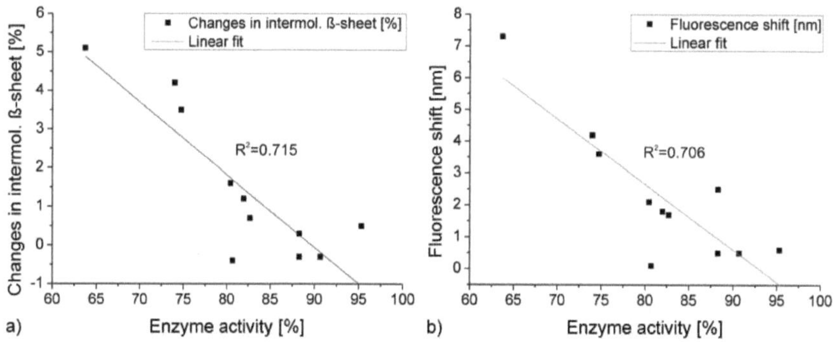

Fig. 6.18: Correlation of a) increasing intermolecular β-sheet and b) shifts of fluorescence maxima with residual a-CT enzyme activity. Results were taken from chapter 6.4.

Stepwise analysis of the SFD process using different proteins and nozzle types yielded the following important pieces of information:

First, no general assumptions can be made for the stability of unknown proteins during spray-freeze-drying. a-CT and HSA, originally selected due to the differences in their secondary structure, reacted very differently to the stresses presented by atomization, freezing and subsequent freeze-drying. While α-chymotrypsin stability was substantially affected during some processing steps, changes to HSA were mostly within the limits of error. Hence, the protein itself seems to have an important influence on the outcome of the SFD process.

Second, the concentration of the protein solution was an important factor. 100 mg/mL a-CT solutions were much more susceptible to atomization and freeze-drying than a-CT at a concentration of 10 mg/mL. According to the excluded volume theory, conformational stability should increase at high concentrations, while colloidal stability (e.g. aversion of aggregation) should decrease at the same time [Minton 1997]. Guo et al. [2006] additionally stated that protein stability at high concentrations is protein-dependent because other factors like protein-protein interactions, protein dynamics and solvent effects come into play. In SFD however, low solid contents are not always feasible because the resulting products do not consist of distinct, spherical particles. The problem becomes even more complex if powders are intended for needle-free ballistic injection where superior particle stability and density, which are necessary to penetrate the skin, and a high protein load are crucial [Kendall et al. 2004; Ziegler 2006].

Third, protein damage during atomization is partially reversed by quench freezing. Results in this thesis further indicated that proteins underwent slight refolding during quench-freezing. As only little increases in intermolecular β-sheet and λ_{max} values were detected, no simultaneous formation of aggregates is suspected.

Fourth, the choice of the nozzle had an important effect on protein denaturation. Especially the 25 kHz (and to a lesser extent the 120 kHz) design inflicted higher degrees of damage than the other nozzles. Additionally, results often showed stronger deviations if high damage was induced to a-CT during an atomization or SFD experiment. This suggests higher inhomogeneity in atomization under certain circumstances. As adsorption at the air/liquid interface cannot be the only reason for loss in activity and native structure, other parameters like increasing temperatures or the occurrence of cavitation could further reduce protein stability. The influence of those factors is investigated in the following chapter.

7. Characterization of ultrasonic nozzles

7.1 Introduction

As the choice of nozzle proved to be a critical factor in producing stable protein particles (see chapter 6), it was necessary to gain further insight in potential stress factors during liquid atomization. The two-fluid nozzle was not included in the experimental design as it showed inferior feasibility during the SFD experiments. First, liquid feed homogeneity was evaluated, to obtain more details about the pulsation of different pumps at various feed rates. Second, particle size distributions at different atomization frequencies at a liquid feed rate of 1 mL/min were evaluated. For this task, a 200 mg/mL placebo formulation was used containing trehalose, mannitol and dextran (MW=10 kDa) at a mass ration of 3:3:4 ("TMD 334"). As size distribution of the fine droplet spray is to be preserved in the final particles, conclusions on actual droplet size and surface area during the spraying step should be possible [Sonner 2002]. Then, temperature profiles at different power settings and nozzle frequencies were recorded to allow estimation of protein stress due to heat dissipation. Finally, the occurrence of cavitation was determined by sonochemical methods, using potassium iodide, ammonium iron (II) sulfate hexahydrate and terephthalic acid as marker solutions.

7.2 Homogeneity of liquid feed rate

Fluctuations in feed homogeneity can affect the particle size distribution and therefore should be considered a critical parameter during the atomization step [Sonner 2002]. Three different pump systems were evaluated in this thesis, possibly exhibiting different levels of pulsation: a Microchem rotary pump (KSB AG, Frankenthal, Germany), a Pharmacia Biotech P-1 peristaltic pump bearing 6 rollers (Amersham Pharmacia Biotech Inc, Piscataway, USA) and a Ismatec ISM597D peristaltic pump with 10 rollers (Ismatec SA, Glattbrugg, Switzerland). Fig. 7.1 shows the liquid feed rate versus time profile recorded by the Proline Promass 83A coriolis mass flow unit (Endress+Hauser

GmbH+Co. KG, Weil am Rhein, Germany) with and without activated atomization. The sdv values of the individual graphs were used to objectively assess the fluctuations in the feed rate/time profile.

Due to its way of operation, the rotary pump is supposed to deliver an essentially oscillation-free liquid feed suited perfectly for generating particles with a narrow span under reproducible atomization conditions [KSB 2009]. However, two drawbacks negatively affected the feasibility of this pump design. First, the dead volume of the pump chamber was 5 mL. This is disadvantageous for laboratory scale experiments as comparably large quantities of mostly expensive protein formulations become necessary. Due to this reason, the rotary pump was not applied for the standard enzyme preparations in chapter 6. Second, the investigated liquid feed rates were very low for this pump design, leading to long time intervals until steady state feed rates were achieved. According to the manufacturer, comparably high flow resistances and liquid feed rates are required to quickly achieve reproducible and steady flow rates using this rotary pump [KSB 2009]. Therefore, the tube diameter was artificially reduced by applying a hose clip between pump and nozzle. Additionally, the rotary pump could be operated in automatic mode where the performance was gauged by the actual liquid feed rate. These steps substantially reduced fluctuations of the liquid feed, leading to sdv values comparable to the peristaltic pumps (Table 7.1).

The peristaltic pumps, on the other hand, showed very good handling from the start, especially for the low volume formulations. Feed homogeneity was independent of the actual liquid feed rate and benefited slightly from the change from six to ten rollers. As soon as atomization was turned on, fluctuations of the liquid feed rate increased for all pumps which is noticeable by higher sdv values (Table 7.1). This could possibly be caused by a higher flow resistance inside the nozzle due to the vibration of the piezoelectric crystal.

In summary, all pump systems showed good performance for the investigated feed rates. Surprisingly, the rotary pump was not able to outperform the peristaltic pump designs at the given experimental settings. The very low volumes and liquid feed rates required during laboratory scale SFD seemed to favor a classic peristaltic pump designs as handling was far more easily. If larger volumes and/or feed rates are needed (as e.g. during scale-up), the feasibility of the rotary pump could improve substantially. The pulsation effects are expected to decrease even further with increasing feed rates and the above described problems should become less relevant. At the low liquid feed rate of 1 mL/min, however, only little influence of the choice of pump should be expected on the particle size distribution.

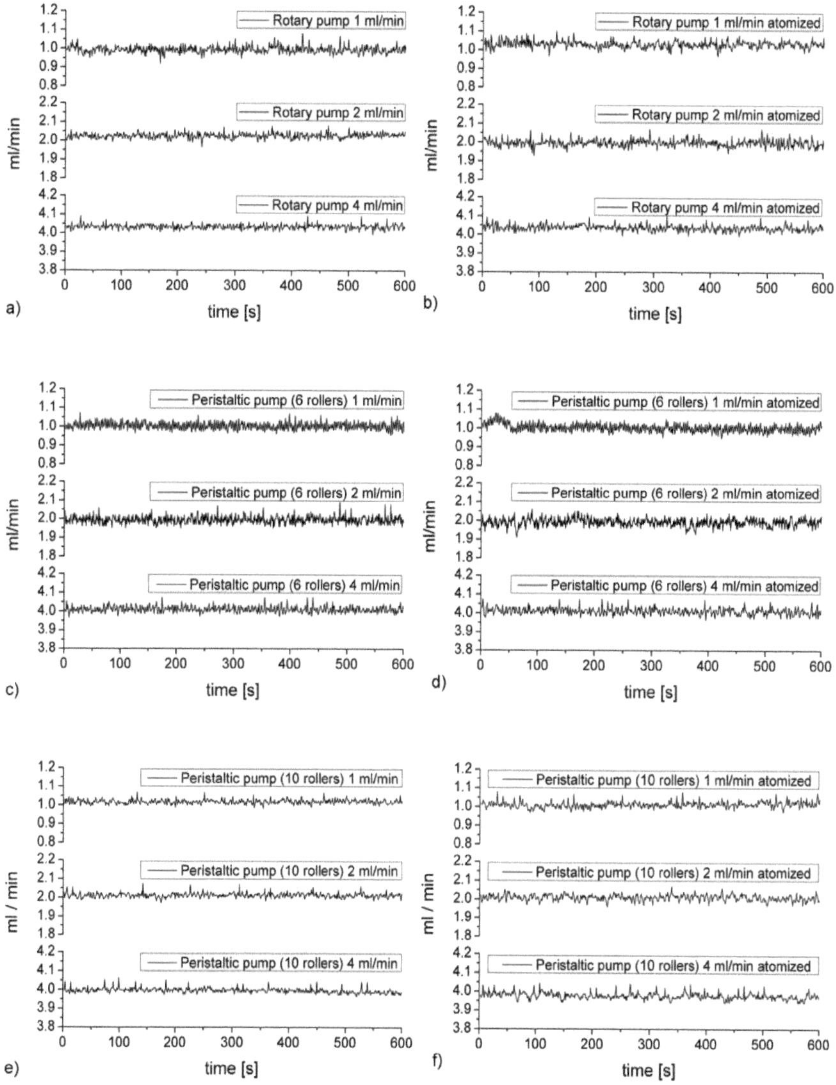

Fig. 7.1: Flow homogeneity of different pumps with and without atomization determined by a Promass 83A coriolis mass flow measuring system. a)+b) Rotary pump, c)+d) Peristaltic pump with 6 rollers, e)+f) Peristaltic pump with 10 rollers.

Table 7.1: Standard deviations of the liquid feed/time profile of different pump systems with and without atomization.

	1 mL/min	2 mL/min	4 mL/min
sdv rotary pump	0.019	0.014	0.013
sdv rotary pump atomized	0.019	0.019	0.015
sdv peristaltic pump (6 rollers)	0.020	0.022	0.018
sdv peristaltic pump (6 rollers) atomized	0.022	0.023	0.019
sdv peristaltic pump (10 rollers)	0.012	0.012	0.012
sdv peristaltic pump (10 rollers) atomized	0.017	0.016	0.017

7.3 Size distribution of SFD particles

Samples for the determination of particle size were generated from a 200 mg/mL TMD 334 placebo formulation that has previously been used for stabilizing proteins during SFD [Maa et al. 2004]. The experiments were performed equal to the SFD process described in chapter 4.3. A power input of 3W in combination with a liquid feed rate of 1 mL/min was used during all experiments.

According to literature, droplets created by an ultrasound nozzle should give a log normal size distribution [Berger 1998]. This could be observed for the final SFD particles in this work, supporting the theory that the distribution of the droplets is preserved during the freeze-drying step (Fig. 7.2a).

In many cases however, evaluation of the SFD products by laser diffraction revealed bimodal particle size distributions after initial dispersion in acetone. The first (strong) signal lay roughly between 10 μm and 100 μm while the second (weaker) signal could be detected between 200 μm and 500 μm (data not shown). As the intensity of the second peak was strongly reduced after 10 min of stirring, it obviously consisted of mostly agglomerates that could be dissipated over time. The existence of agglomerates was also confirmed by the SEM pictures presented in Fig. 7.2b and c, while Fig. 7.2d appeared to be mostly free of aggregates. In most cases a monomodal particle distribution could be achieved after 10 min, but sometimes the second signal was still detectable and had to be assigned to exceptionally large particles.

Evaluation of PSD was performed using the data recorded after 10 min to reduce bias towards larger particle sizes by aggregates. The resulting graphs were analyzed by calculating volume mean diameter, $d_{v,50}$, and $span_v$. This led to deviating results as soon as a bimodal particle size distribution was present. In Fig. 7.2a, for example, comparable results should be expected considering the close match of all three graphs. However, this is only true for results of the rotary and the peristaltic pump (6 rollers), giving a volume mean diameter of 41 µm and 42 µm, respectively.

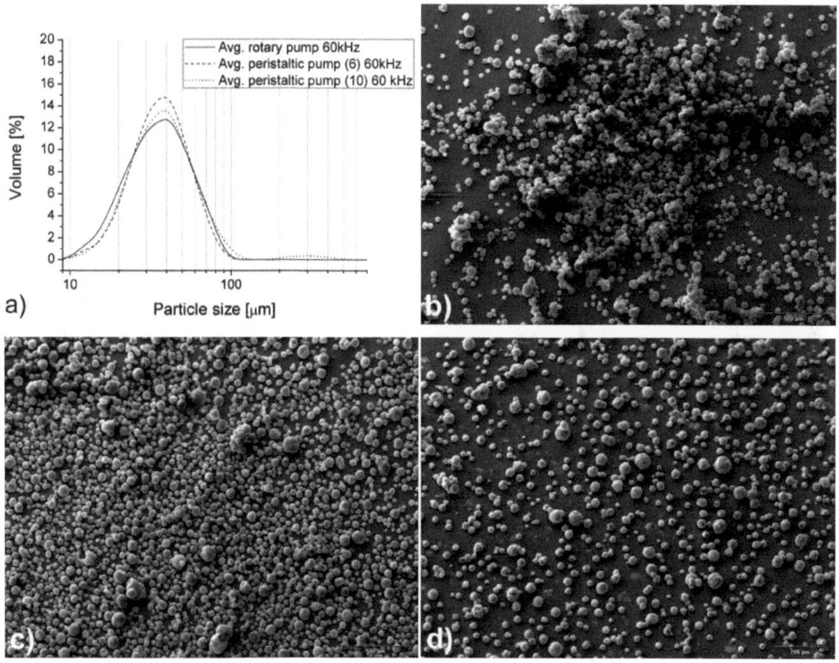

Fig. 7.2: a) PSD measured by laser diffraction, b) - d) SEM pictures of SFD particles atomized at 60 kHz and forwarded by a peristaltic pump with 6 rollers (50x), a peristaltic pump with 10 rollers (50x) and a rotary pump pump (100x), respectively.

The Ismatec peristaltic pump, showing a weak second peak at around 300 µm, produced a mean volume diameter of 54.48 µm. This result is implausible, considering that the same nozzle was used in all three experiments. Similar deviations could be observed for $d_{v,50}$ (39 vs. 47 µm) and $span_v$ (1.033 vs. 1.196). If PSDs deviated noticeably, like in Fig. 7.3a, differences became even stronger, resulting in very high mean volume diameters of up to 64 µm for the 48 kHz nozzle.

SEM pictures of the 48 kHz experiments revealed extraordinary large particles for the rotary and peristaltic pump (6 rollers) that biased the above mentioned evaluation methods (Fig. 7.3b+d). Therefore particle characterization using the mode of the strongest peak seemed more promising. On the other hand, this means that $span_v$ values are not available anymore for evaluating differences between the pump systems. Still, this method of evaluation was the only way to objectively compare results from the individual experiments.

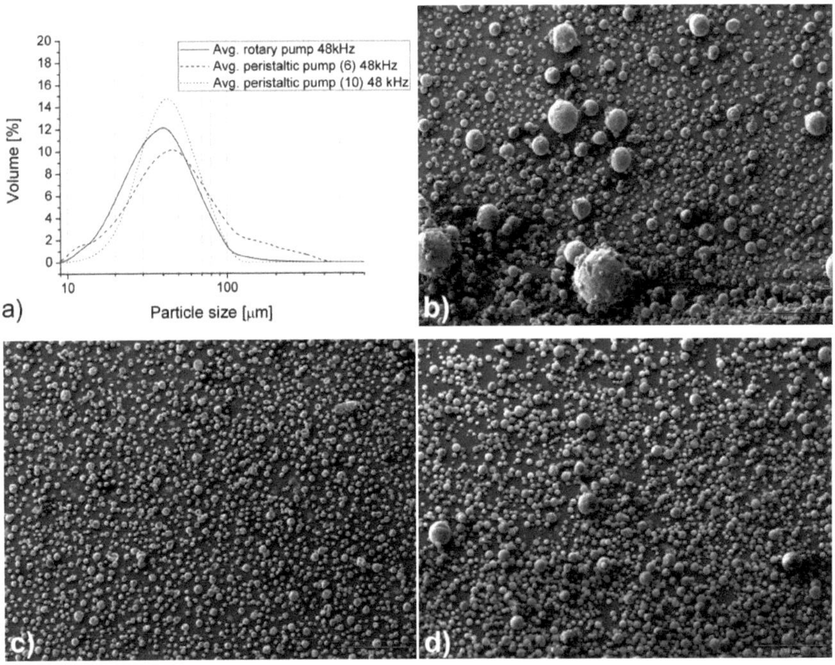

Fig. 7.3: a) PSD measured by laser diffraction, b)-d) SEM pictures of SFD particles atomized at 48 kHz and forwarded by a peristaltic pump with 6 rollers, a peristaltic pump with 10 rollers and a rotary pump, respectively (all 50x magnification).

The earlier-mentioned correlation between increasing nozzle frequency and decreasing particle size is once more visible in Fig. 7.4. Diameters ranged from 52 µm (25 kHz) to 30 µm (120 kHz) depending on the nozzle type used. Results from particles sprayed at same nozzle frequency were pretty close for most of the pump systems investigated. Only atomization by the 25 kHz nozzle showed noticeable deviations between the rotary pump (46 µm ± 1 µm) and the peristaltic pumps with either 6 rollers (52 µm ± 2 µm) or 10 rollers (51.1 µm ± 1.3 µm). On the other hand, results for the 60 kHz experiments were almost identical. No correlation could be found between pump systems and the resulting particle homogeneity. However, formation of the exceptionally large droplet fraction was mainly observed when using low frequency nozzles (25 kHz and 48 kHz) for atomization.

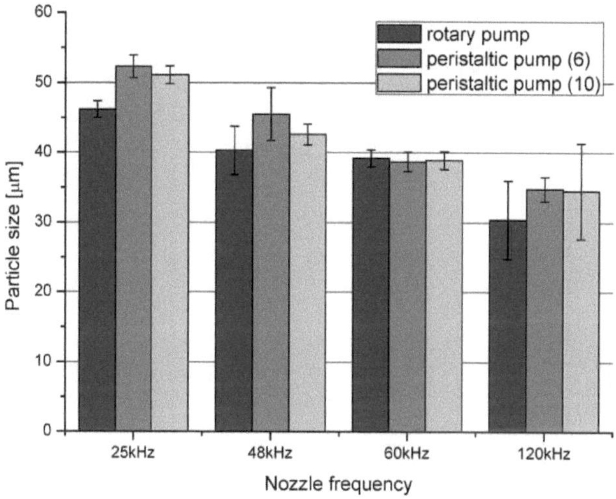

Fig. 7.4: Particle diameters determined by the mode value of the highest peak within the PSDs.

7.3.1 Overall comparison and discussion

Increasing nozzle frequencies led to smaller SFD particles visible by the decrease in main particle diameter from 52 µm to 30 µm. The range of possible particle sizes was noticeably narrower compared to the results determined for pure water by [Sono-Tek 2009] (between 20 µm and 65 µm). As the 200 mg/mL TMD 334 solution exhibits substantial differences to water in rheologic properties (e.g. viscosity, density, surface tension, etc.), these findings were not surprising.

The extraordinary large droplets between 200 µm and 500 µm were far beyond the fine droplet spray usually generated by these ultrasound nozzles. However, their existence could definitely be verified by the SEM pictures as well as the PSDs presented in Fig. 7.3. The most plausible explanation is that a fraction of the droplets experienced coalescence during their descend through the vapor phase. Alternatively, the droplets could also have converged after hitting the wall of the bowl rather than the surface of the cryogen. This would be especially important for the 25 kHz and 48 kHz nozzles as their droplet clouds exhibited a relatively wide spray diameter.

The pump system employed for delivering the liquid feed had no measurable effect on particle size distribution at the examined conditions. Within certain limits, the ultrasonic nozzles were able to deliver comparable droplets size distributions irrespective of the pumping system used. Furthermore, pulsations determined for peristaltic pumps in chapter 7.2 were only slightly worse than for the rotary pump. Hence, the choice of pump should be based on its feasibility which means that peristaltic pumps should work fine for laboratory scale SFD using small volumes and low liquid feed rates. Rotary pumps could become valuable if sample volume and liquid feed rate increase during scale-up.

7.4 Temperature measurements

7.4.1 25 kHz nozzle

For the 25 kHz nozzle, atomization could already be achieved at comparably low power input, and therefore temperature measurements were only conducted at 1W, 2W and 3W. Higher settings were not examined as they would unlikely be applied during a standard SFD run since they would cause unnecessary protein stress (see temperature measurements in this chapter as well as the investigation of cavitation in section 7.5). Increasing the atomization power led to elevated temperatures of the spray cloud. While 1W power input increased the temperature from 22°C to 31°C after 12 min (ΔT +9°C), 2W and 3W led to steady-state temperatures of 39°C (ΔT +17°C) and 46°C (ΔT +24°C), respectively. Surprisingly, the temperature-time-profiles showed obvious fluctuations of up to 2°C between two measurement points (recording interval: 5s) (Fig. 7.5a). These variations occurred during the entire recorded process and were independent from the applied atomizing power input. Compared to higher frequency nozzles the 25 kHz design led to the lowest ΔT values, indicating only minor thermal stress for proteins.

7.4.2 48 kHz nozzle

The 48 kHz nozzle was set to power levels of 3W, 6W and 9W during the following experiments as settings below 3W resulted in incomplete atomization. This was noticeable by the formation of very large droplets accompanied by temporary sputtering of the nozzle. According to the manufacturer, atomizing power usually lies between 1W and 15W, so the chosen values were still considered appropriate [Sono-Tek 2009]. Surprisingly, temperatures determined at 3W lay around 32.5°C (ΔT +10.5°C) which is substantially lower than the readings from the 25 kHz nozzle at the same power input. As higher frequencies usually create higher heat dissipation, an increase in temperature was suspected. However, any readings from the 25 kHz nozzle were surpassed by further increasing the atomizing power. Droplet temperatures increased to 50°C at 6W (ΔT +28°C) and 64°C at 9W (ΔT +42°C), respectively (Fig. 7.5b). The temperature-time-profile showed fluctuations of 2°C at 3W and 6W which was comparable to the 25 kHz nozzle. Interestingly, the profile became more unsteady at a power level of 9W where sudden temperature changes of up to 4°C were measured.

7.4.3 60 kHz nozzle

The trend to higher spray temperatures for higher nozzle frequencies was continued with the 60 kHz design. By increasing the power input from 3W to 6W and 9W, steady state temperatures of 38°C (ΔT +16°C), 58°C (ΔT +36°C) and 69°C (ΔT +47°C) were achieved, respectively (Fig. 7.5c). Surprisingly, low fluctuations of 1°C were measured if atomization was performed at a power level of 3W. Higher setting increased fluctuations again up to 3°C at 9W which still indicated superior spray homogeneity in comparison to the 48 kHz nozzle. Temperatures at 3W were again slightly lower than values determined for the 25 kHz nozzle, but the difference was further reduced to 8°C.

7.4.4 120 kHz nozzle

The 120 kHz nozzle reached the highest overall steady-state temperatures. At 3W power input, temperatures rose to 44°C (ΔT +22°C), which was equivalent to the heat generated by the 25 kHz nozzle at the same settings. Increasing the power level to 6W and 9W resulted in substantially higher temperature readings of 64°C (ΔT +42°C) and 80°C (ΔT +58°C) after 12 minutes, respectively (Fig. 7.5d). Interestingly, the profile for atomization at 3W was comparable to the other nozzles, showing only fluctuations of approximately 2°C. By increasing the power level to 6W and 9W, the profile became much more unstable exhibiting temperature changes up to 13°C. In addition, the appearance of small air bubbles at the connection between nozzle and tube could be observed during atomization at 9W. Possible reasons for the occurrence of the air bubbles are discussed in the following section.

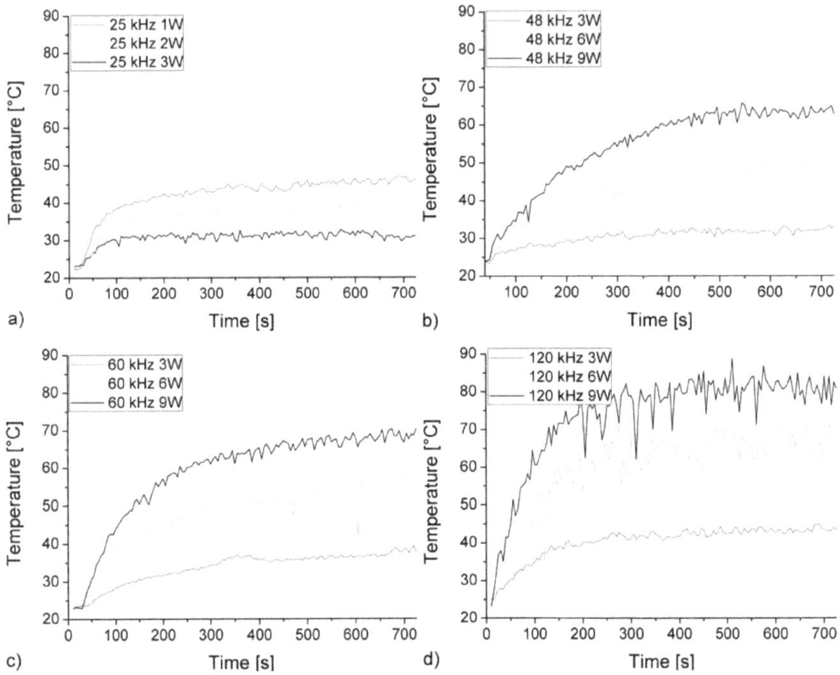

Fig. 7.5: Temperature over time profile of the a) 25 kHz, b) 48 kHz, c) 60 kHz and d) 120 kHz nozzle. The profile of the 120 kHz nozzle showed noticeable fluctuations at 6W and 9W.

7.4.5 Overall comparison and discussion

In Fig. 7.6, the steady-state temperatures of the different nozzles are plotted against the applied power input. With increasing nozzle frequency and atomization power, augmented heat dissipation was produced. Regression analysis revealed R^2 values of 0.999 (25 kHz), 0.989 (48 kHz), 0.954 (60 kHz) and 0.995 (120 kHz), indicating a very close linear relationship within the investigated range. The 25 kHz nozzle deviated from its higher frequency counterparts, as it already showed atomization at 1W power input and exhibited differences in its temperature profiles. Lowest temperatures could be achieved using the 25 kHz nozzle, followed by the 48 kHz, 60 kHz and 120 kHz models. The surprisingly high temperatures of the spray cloud at 25 kHz and 3W were probably caused by the outer hull of the nozzle. This extra layer around the nozzle horn serves as a barrier against the ambient temperature, thereby insulating the nozzle (Fig. 7.7).

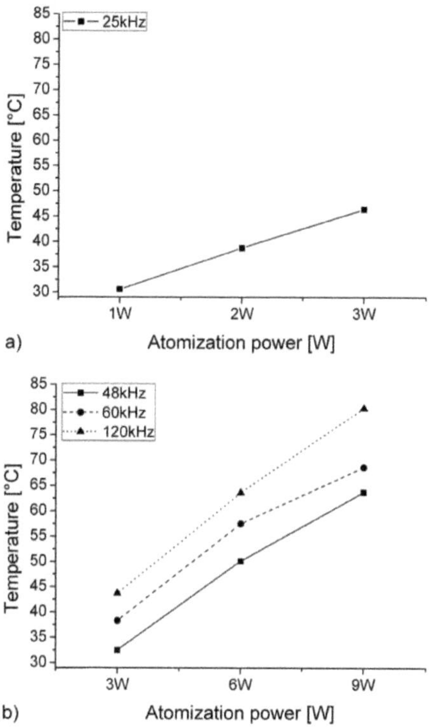

Fig. 7.6: Comparison of the steady-state temperatures of four ultrasonic nozzles using different power input levels. a) 25kHz nozzle, b) 48kHz, 60kHz and 120kHz nozzles.

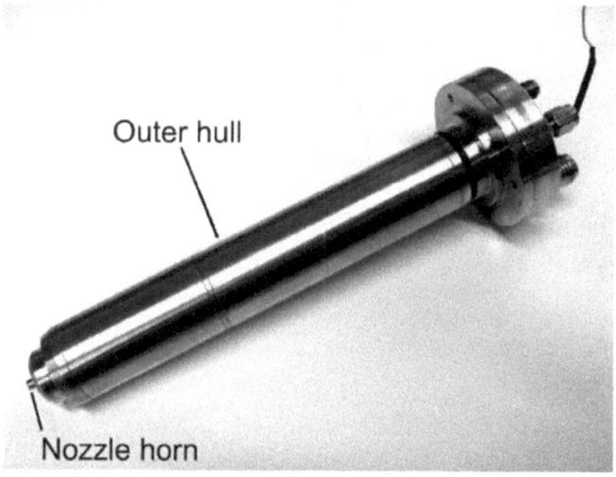

Fig. 7.7: Picture of the 25 kHz nozzle, showing the tip of the nozzle horn surrounded by its outer hull.

A possible linear relationship between nozzle temperature and residual enzyme activity was evaluated as well. For this task, results from the atomization experiments performed with the 100 mg/mL a-CT solutions (see chapter 6.4.1) were plotted against the steady state nozzle temperatures at 3W power input. However, no correlation could be determined for the investigated settings (data not shown). A reason could be that the power input of 3W in combination with the short duration of the spraying step (usually 2-3 minutes) was insufficient to reach temperatures that were critical for the protein. Alternatively, either cavitation alone or cavitation together with nozzle temperature could also be responsible for the protein damage determined in chapter 6.4.1.

It is important to note that temperature measurements were performed at the tip of the nozzle, but the thermally relevant oscillation of the piezoelectric crystal is located further inside the nozzle body [Sono-Tek 2009]. Therefore, thermal stress may have been even higher than indicated from this experimental setup. The appearance of air bubbles at the connection between nozzle and tube during longer atomization periods (see chapter 7.4.4) could easily be explained if temperatures actually reached the boiling point at the inside. This would imply a temperature gradient of at least 20°C between piezoelectric crystal and the position of the thermocouple which seems high but still possible – especially for high temperatures at the outlet. Those considerations should be taken into account when choosing an ultrasound nozzle for atomization of heat-susceptible proteins.

Finally, noticeable differences in fluctuation intensity of the temperature-time-profiles could be determined depending on the nozzle frequency and the atomizing conditions. Deviations were especially high using the 120 kHz nozzle at 9W which caused severe temperature fluctuations of up to 13°C. One possible reason would be that the number of droplets per time interval that hit the measurement point varied, which led to differences in the heat transferred to the thermocouple. However, variations would have to be rather intense if they caused these large declines in temperature. Pulsations determined for the liquid feed were too low to be responsible, and as the sensor was placed directly beneath the nozzle orifice it seems unlikely that major parts of the droplet fraction were not included during the measurement. Alternatively, the temperature of the droplet spray could have actually varied. If atomization power exceeds a certain threshold cavitation effects occur, literally ripping the solution apart. As a result, large "chunks" of fluid are ejected [Sono-Tek 2009] that could exhibit noticeable differences in temperature. This process could have been further augmented by pulsations in the liquid feed rate. Additionally, the oscillation and subsequent collapse of gas bubbles during cavitation [Sponer 1990] could also have led the observed air bubbles at the connection between nozzle and tube, and therefore cavitation should be considered the most likely cause for the above described deviations.

7.5 Cavitation measurements

Protein damage by different ultrasonic nozzles, as described in chapter 6, cannot be explained by elevated temperatures alone. The 25 kHz nozzle, for example, caused only minor increases in temperature, but induced massive damage to a-CT at high concentrations. As described in chapter 4.4.2, rapid collapse of small air bubbles during atomization could have led to the generation of free radicals by cavitation. This presents a possible destabilization pathway for proteins by chemical denaturation [Riesz et al. 1992; van de Weert et al. 2000]. Therefore, the generation of free radicals by cavitation was quantified. Potassium iodide (KI), ammonium iron(II) sulfate hexahydrate (Fe) and terephthalic acid (TA) solutions were prepared in accordance to chapter 4.4.2. The feasibility of the experimental setup was assessed by preliminary experiments using an ultrasonic bath and an ultrasonic homogenizer. Evaluation of the spraying step itself showed very poor reproducibility if performed equal to the SFD experiments in chapter 6. Therefore, the experimental setup had to be redesigned for cavitation analysis as described in section 4.4.2.

7.5.1 Preliminary experiments

Ultrasonic bath

First, the generation of free radicals in an ultrasonic bath (Bandelin electronic GmbH & Co. KG, Germany) was observed. The apparatus had an operational frequency of 35 kHz and applied an ultrasonic power of 120 W. Samples were taken every 10 minutes, and changes in absorbance or fluorescence were quantified.

As can be seen in Fig. 7.8, only slight effects were visible over time, showing minimal, but steady increase of radicals with continuing exposure. Analysis by fluorescence spectroscopy showed highest sensitivity, as intensity increased on average by 6 AU per 10 minutes. Changes in absorbance were relatively low for KI and Fe resulting in a mean incline of 0.002 units/10 min and 0.001 units/10 min, respectively. Therefore, it seems that the high overall ultrasonic power of 120 W was dispersed within the 4 litres tank of the water bath, resulting in only minor oxidation due to cavitation.

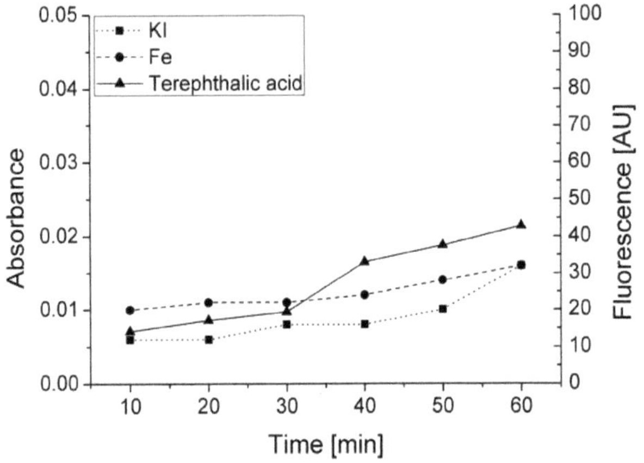

Fig. 7.8: Quantification of ultrasonic-induced cavitation by oxidation of KI, Fe and TA over time (ultrasonic bath).

Ultrasonic homogenizer

Then, effects on KI, Fe and TA due to ultrasonic homogenization were evaluated with help of a Bransonic sonifier (Branson ultrasonic Corp., Danbury, USA), using the power input level 7 (non-dimensional value). The tip of the homogenizer lance was placed inside a beaker containing the reagent solution and set to continuous operation. To compensate for the heat generated during sonication the beaker was surrounded by ice (Fig. 7.9). Comparable to the experiments conducted in the ultrasonic bath, samples were taken every 10 minutes and subsequently analyzed.

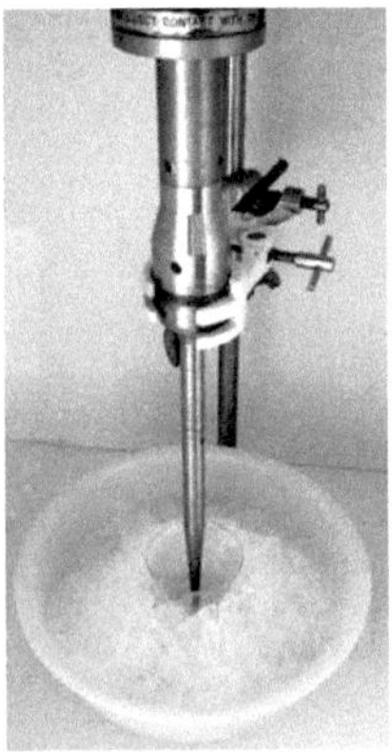

Fig. 7.9: Experimental setup for the ultrasonic homogenizer

The results from the ultrasonic homogenizer indicated elevated oxidation stress induced by cavitation. Again, fluorescence spectroscopy was the most sensitive quantification method, increasing on average by 112 AU within 10 minutes. A strong signal could also be detected for KI, showing an average rise in absorbance by 0.05 units/10 min. However, measurements using Fe only gave slight increases in absorbance (+0.01 units/10 min) (Fig. 7.10). By setting the mean inclines of the ultrasonic bath and the homogenizer into relation, one can see that the homogenizer induced between 19 (TA) and 25 times (KI) more cavitation than the ultrasonic bath. Results for Fe were lower, indicating only a 10 times higher increase in absorbance by the homogenizer. However, as Fe values determined for the ultrasound bath were near the limits of detection, those results were prone to noise.

Based on the results obtained by the preliminary experiments, measuring the oxidation by KI, Fe and terephthalic acid solutions seemed to be a feasible way for the quantification of cavitation effects.

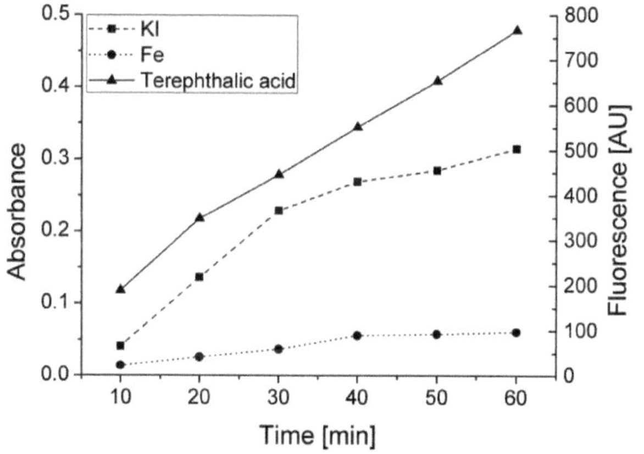

Fig. 7.10: Quantification of ultrasonic-induced cavitation by oxidation of KI, Fe and TA over time (ultrasonic homogenizer).

7.5.2 Nozzle-induced cavitation

Feasibility of the nozzle experiments was reduced by the fact that the vibrations of the nozzle tip were impeded if immersed deeply into the reagent solutions. This led to incomplete atomization or no atomization at all, accompanied by an error signal of the broadband generator controlling the nozzle. By placing the orifice right below the surface of the solution, the 48 kHz, 60 kHz and 120 kHz nozzles could still be operated at the desired power inputs. The 25 kHz nozzle was not able to achieve continuous atomization, possibly due to its short spray tip, and gave an error signal or showed severe sputtering during operation. Changes in nozzle placement or increases of the power input beyond 3W did not lead to any improvements. Therefore, cavitation by the 25 kHz nozzle design could not be evaluated. This is highly disadvantageous as the elevated protein damage after spraying at 25 kHz (see chapter 6) could not be explained by the low nozzle temperatures determined in chapter 7.4. Therefore, the occurrence of cavitation would have been a plausible reason for the above mentioned results.

Terephthalic acid

Plotting the fluorescence intensity against increasing power input showed a nearly linear relationship for the 48 kHz and 60 kHz nozzles (Fig. 7.11). Spraying with the 60 kHz nozzle resulted in relatively low increases in fluorescence, irrespective of the power input applied. However, cavitation effects increased substantial for the 48 kHz and 120 kHz nozzles. Increasing the power input from 6W to 9W at 120 kHz lead to reduced reproducibility, noticeable by the high standard deviation (Table 7.2). Additionally, the last measurement point deviated noticeably from the other measurements, indicating an almost exponential increase in cavitation. This inhomogeneity is similar to the increased fluctuations in temperature at 9W determined in chapter 7.4.

Table 7.2: Fluorescence intensity of oxidized terephthalic acid after atomization by different nozzles.

Power input	48 kHz [AU]	sdv	60 kHz [AU]	sdv	120 kHz [AU]	sdv
3W	63	4.562	24	6.272	121	25.497
6W	115	15.983	39	11.343	249	16.825
9W	179	31.073	67	7.447	505	109.463

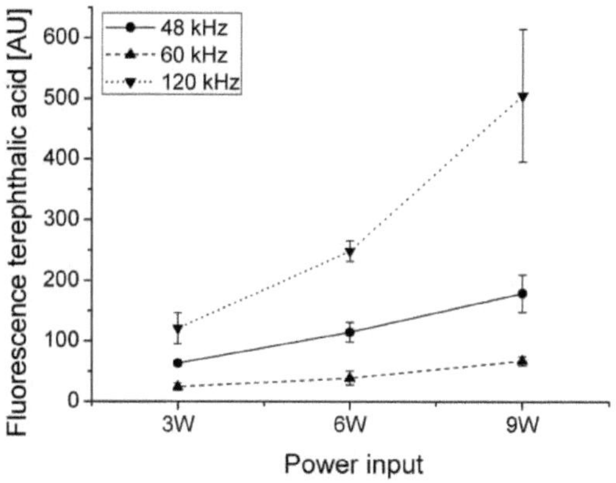

Fig. 7.11: Correlation between atomization power and fluorescence intensity after oxidation of TA by free radicals due to cavitation.

Overall fluorescence intensities of the 60 kHz nozzle were at very low levels, comparable to results determined from preliminary experiments using the ultrasonic bath. The 48 kHz nozzle delivered roughly three times as much damage as its 60 kHz counterpart, while the 120 kHz design inflicted highest cavitation effects. For this nozzle, atomization stress - especially at 6W and 9W - nearly equaled oxidation after ultrasonic homogenization which was quite excessive.

Potassium Iodide

Oxidation of KI due to the appearance of cavitation led to findings comparable to the terephthalic acid experiments. The 60 kHz nozzle showed lowest cavitation effects with an increase in absorbance by 0.045 units at most. Oxidation of the KI solution atomized at 48 kHz was increased substantially (by factors between 2x and 4x), while the 120 kHz nozzle caused the by far highest increases in absorbance, reaching values up to 0.343 (Table 7.3). Standard deviations were mostly low except for the numbers determined at 120 kHz, especially at 9W. This last data point also deviated from a possible linear relationship. In contrast to the fluorescence experiments, however, it still lay within the margin of error (Fig. 7.12).

Comparison with the preliminary experiments indicated that cavitation stress of the 60 kHz nozzle was again close to the damage inflicted by the ultrasonic bath. The 48 kHz nozzle yielded slightly elevated oxidative effects, while results from the 120 kHz design were again highest and resembled the extreme damage induced by the ultrasonic homogenizer.

Table 7.3: Absorbance of the KI solution after atomization by different nozzle types.

Power input	48 kHz [A]	sdv	60 kHz [A]	sdv	120 kHz [A]	sdv
3W	0.042	0.005	0.01	0.002	0.133	0.018
6W	0.08	0.003	0.026	0.004	0.209	0.023
9W	0.093	0.003	0.045	0.009	0.343	0.089

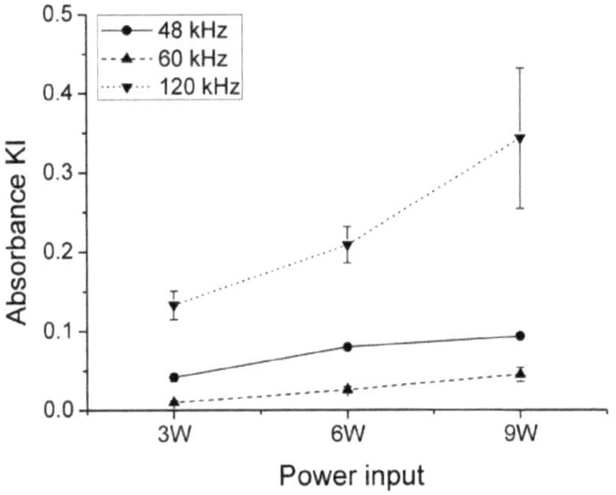

Fig. 7.12: Relationship between atomization power and absorbance of the KI solution after oxidation by free radicals due to cavitation.

Ammonium iron(II) sulfate hexahydrate

Results from the experiments using TA and KI as marker solutions were supported by the evaluation of Fe oxidation. Again, the 60 kHz nozzle showed the lowest oxidation effects, exhibiting increases of maximal 0.013 units at 9W, followed by the 48 kHz nozzle and the 120 kHz nozzle topping out at highest values (Fig. 7.13). Standard deviations were pretty close except for atomization at 120 kHz (see Table 7.4). Here, the results from spraying with the 120 kHz nozzle using 6W atomization power showed even higher fluctuations than at 9W. In contrast to KI and TA a linear relationship is retained through all performed experiments.

Table 7.4: Absorbance of Fe after atomization by different nozzle types.

Power input	48 kHz [A]	sdv	60 kHz [A]	sdv	120 kHz [A]	sdv
3W	0.011	0.003	0.003	0.001	0.023	0.009
6W	0.019	0.006	0.006	0.004	0.054	0.021
9W	0.026	0.007	0.013	0.004	0.082	0.012

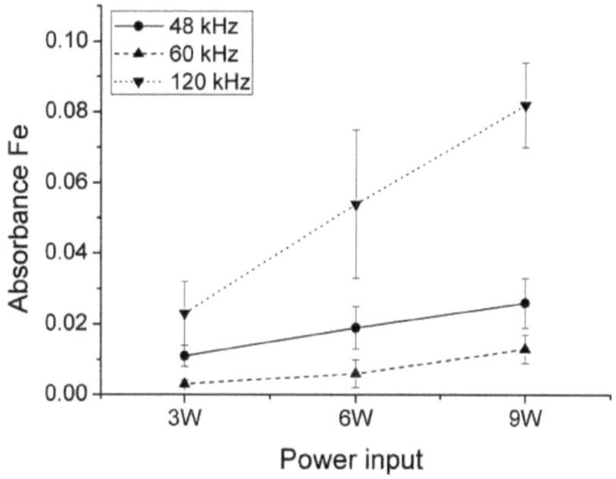

Fig. 7.13: Absorbance versus power input plot of an in-situ oxidized Fe solution after atomization in different nozzles.

7.5.3 Overall comparison and discussion

Experiments performed in this chapter clearly indicated that the occurrence of cavitation can present additional stress to proteins during SFD. Highest sensitivity for the quantification of cavitation was achieved by measuring increases in fluorescence intensity of terephthalic acid after oxidation. Changes in absorbance of KI/I_2 were less pronounced but still noticeable, while results from the oxidation of Fe were partially near the limit of detection.

Reproducibility of the evaluation was increased by immersing the nozzles into the reagent solutions during operation. A possible reason for the improvements over the standard experimental SFD setup could be that during the spraying process the fine fraction of the droplets was carried away, making it impossible to quantitatively evaluate the appearance of cavitation. This is especially important, as the same effect could occur during standard SFD experiments (even though it should be less pronounced for ultrasound nozzles than previously described for two-fluid atomization – see chapter 6.6). Depending on the question if protein damage differs substantially within the fine droplet fraction, this observation could strongly influence overall evaluations. However, those investigations lie beyond the scope of this work, but should be considered in the future.

From the nozzles investigated, the 120 kHz type was able to induce the highest degree of oxidative effects to any of the reagent solutions used. It is interesting to see that no direct relation between nozzle frequency and cavitation intensity can be deducted, as the 120 kHz nozzle was followed by its 48 kHz counterpart in every experiment. The 60 kHz nozzle seemed to be the most promising design as it exhibited least oxidation of the reagent solutions. Investgation of the effects of the 25 kHz nozzle was not possible because it could not be operated at the given experimental setup. However, protein damage determined in chapter 6.4 as well as comparably low temperature readings in chapter 7.4 suggested that cavitation could be critical for this nozzle type as well.

Equal to chapter 7.4.5, a possible linear relationship between cavitation and enzyme activity was evaluated by plotting increases in absorbance and fluorescence against residual enzyme activity of the atomized 100 mg/mL a-CT solution (power input 3W). Unlike for the temperature measurements, a moderate correlation could be deducted giving R^2 values between -0.64 (TA) and -0.84 (KI) (graphs not shown). This means that cavitation could present a major part of the protein stress during ultrasound atomization. However, as cavitation could only be quantified for the 48 kHz, 60 kHz and 120 kHz nozzles, the significance of evaluation is rather low. In order to obtain statistically reliable results, further investigations are necessary that correlate enzyme activity with the oxidative effects of cavitation over a wide variety of ultrasound atomization settings. This experimental design, however, lies beyond the scope of this thesis but should be considered in future works.

The high standard deviations determined in this chapter, especially at high atomizing power input, suggested noticeable differences in oxidation from experiment to experiment. In chapters 6.4.1 and

6.4.3, obvious variations in enzyme activity as well as secondary and tertiary structure were detected for the nozzles inducing higher protein damage. Fluctuations during temperature readings at demanding atomization conditions were already discussed in chapter 7.4. Cavitation is dependent on numerous parameters including (amongst others) vapor pressure, surface tension, gas solubility, viscosity, temperature, nozzle frequency and active intermediates within the solution [Shah et al. 1999]. During the atomization step nozzle temperatures rise considerably which directly affect many of the before-mentioned factors. Pulsation of the liquid feed rate probably further complicates the influence of cavitation. If all those findings were connected, inhomogeneities concerning the occurrence of heat and cavitation during protein spray-freeze-drying at high power inputs could present a major problem for the whole process.

8. Preparation of microparticles from protein/excipient mixtures by spray-freeze-drying

The third results section of this thesis covers the stabilization of protein microparticles by the addition of excipients to the formulation. Most of the excipients were chosen for their well-known stabilizing properties according to the preferential exclusion ("cryoprotectants") and water replacement ("lyoprotectants") theories [Wang 1999; Wang 2000].

As can be seen in chapter 6, HSA did not show any substantial changes to neither protein secondary nor tertiary structure during SFD and is furthermore lacking any intrinsic enzyme activity. Offering no potential for further stabilization, it was not included in the following series of experiments. a-CT, on the other hand, could suffer noticeable protein damage if processed at high concentrations and demanding atomization conditions.

Hence, two different experimental setups were chosen for the evaluation of the excipients based on the nozzle investigations performed in chapter 7: the first series of experiments used the 60 kHz nozzle at a power input of 3W. This was considered a conservative SFD setup, because the previously determined temperatures and cavitation effects during the spraying step were rather low. For the aggressive SFD experiments, the solutions were atomized using a 120 kHz nozzle at 9W which was supposed to induce maximum protein damage during the spraying step by heat and cavitation effects. In both cases, the same freeze-drying cycle was applied afterwards, posing an additional stress factor to the enzyme due to the removal of water.

8.1 a-CT microparticles from high concentrated solutions (100 mg/mL): conservative setup - 60 kHz 3W

8.1.1 Stabilization with surface-active excipients

Polysorbat 80 has previously been used in various patents at concentrations between 0.1 mg/mL and 0.5 mg/mL to inhibit protein molecules from adsorbing at the air-liquid interface [Wang 1988]. These concentrations lay about 7 to 35 times above the critical micelle concentration (CMC) of the excipient [Wan et al. 1974], indicating that micelles had already formed inside the solution. In addition, an oriented monolayer of surfactant was also covering the complete air/liquid interface [Porter 1994]. Based on the patents detailed by Wang [1988], the stabilization of a-CT has been evaluated in this work by the addition of polysorbat 80 to the solutions in concentrations of 0.25 mg/mL, 0.5 mg/mL and 1 mg/mL. As both enzyme and emulsifier competitively inhibit each other from reaching the droplet surface, the addition of the surfactant should lead to superior a-CT stability if adsorption plays a key role in protein unfolding [Maa et al. 1998].

As can be seen in Fig. 8.1a, polysorbat 80 was able to reduce damage to a-CT tertiary structure by a small amount. λ_{max} underwent bathochrome shifts between 0.6 nm and 1.1 nm which is still slightly below the wavelength shift determined for the SFD experiment without any excipients (+ 1.7 nm). Interestingly, the highest surfactant concentration showed the lowest stabilizing abilities for protein tertiary structure. As all three concentrations lay far above the CMC, similar levels of stabilization would have been expected. However, results were still pretty close to each other.

a-CT secondary structure was completely preserved during all SFD experiments (Fig. 8.1b). Quantification showed the usual fluctuations of α-helix, intra- and intermolecular β-sheet by 0.5% at the most after the addition of polysorbat 80 (see Table 8.1). Evaluation of the pure chymotrypsin solution indicated increases in intermolecular β-sheet by 0.7% which is not considerably higher. As differences were near the limit of detection, the subtle alterations in protein secondary structure after the addition of surfactants could not be discerned by means of FTIR spectroscopy.

Table 8.1: Changes to a-CT secondary structure after SFD with polysorbat 80 in comparison to the SFD experiment performed without excipients.

Formulation	**α-Helix**	**Intramol. β-sheet**	**Intermol. β-sheet**
a-CT pure 100 mg/mL	-0.6%	+0.6%	+0.7%
+PS80 0.25 mg/mL	+0.1%	-0.5%	+0.1%
+PS80 0.5 mg/mL	±0.0%	±0.0%	+0.2%
+PS80 1.0 mg/mL	-0.2%	+0.5%	±0.0%

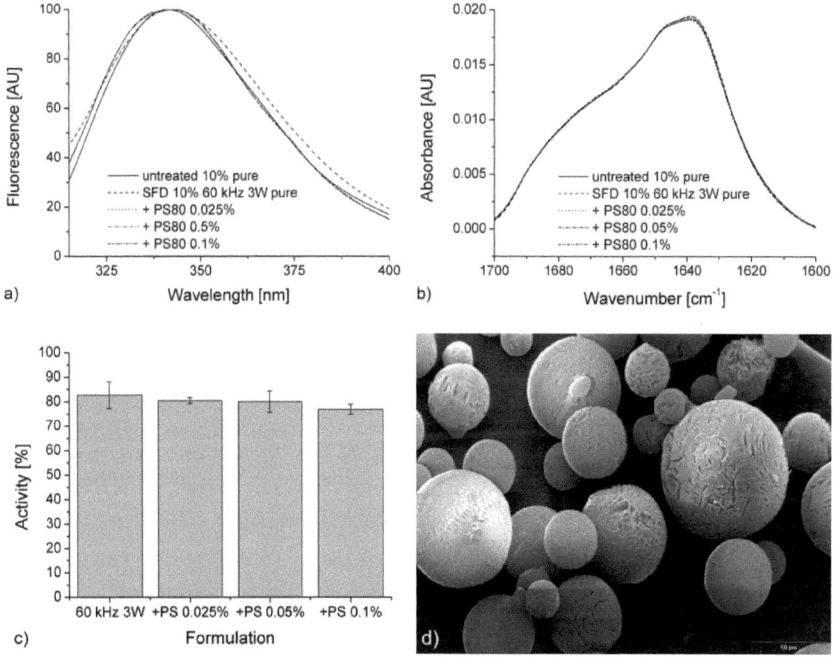

Fig. 8.1: a-CT after SFD at 100 mg/mL using polysorbat 80 as excipient at concentrations of 0.25 mg/mL, 0.5 mg/mL and 1 mg/mL. a) Fluorescence spectra, b) FTIR amide I bands, c) UV activity assay, d) SEM pictures (500x).

Fig. 8.1c displays the a-CT enzyme activity of the pure SFD product and the formulations containing polysorbat 80. Here, no difference in overall protein stability was visible up to 0.5 mg/mL of emulsifier, resulting in residual activities between 82.7% (pure) and 80.1% (+ 0.5 mg/mL polysorbat 80). The protein formulation containing the highest surfactant concentration resulted in slightly inferior a-CT stability of 76.9% which is in accordance to the evaluation of the fluorescence spectra.

SEM pictures revealed no new findings concerning particle morphology (Fig. 8.1d). The concentration of polysorbat 80 seems to be too low to have any microscopic or macroscopic effect. Hence, shape and appearance of the protein particles was not different from the pictures presented in chapter 6.4.3

Considering all results, adsorption of the enzyme at the air-liquid interface seemed to be of subordinate importance for a-CT stability. At the given droplet size no substantial improvements in either secondary structure, tertiary structure or enzyme activity could be detected by the addition of polysorbat 80. This is in concurrence with the results presented in chapter 6 where no correlation between protein damage and droplet surface area at different ultrasound frequencies was observed.

8.1.2 Stabilization with sugars

Sugars (and other polyols) are thoroughly investigated cryo- and lyoprotectants that are often used in classic freeze-drying as they can stabilize proteins during both freezing and subsequent dehydration [Allison et al. 1999; Johnson et al. 2002; Luthra et al. 2007]. As stated by Costantino [2004], a mass ratio of at least 1:1 (protein:sugar) is necessary to ensure full stabilizing potential. In this thesis a mass ratio of 1:2 (protein:sugar) was applied, thus combining good protein stabilization with increased particle rigidity [Maa et al. 2004]. If damage to a-CT would be induced by freezing or the removal of water, then the addition of sucrose or trehalose should result in elevated enzyme stability.

Fig. 8.2a shows the fluorescence spectra of untreated a-CT and of the reconstituted particles generated with and without excipients. The noticeable bathochrome shift of λ_{max} by 1.7 nm for SFD of the pure enzyme solution was completely averted by the addition of the sugars. The fluorescence maximum for the trehalose formulation laid even slightly below results of untreated a-CT (-0.2 nm). Hence, no damage to protein tertiary structure could be determined.

Comparison of the individual amide I bands of untreated and processed samples revealed subtle differences in protein secondary structure (Fig. 8.2b). The small increase in intermolecular β-sheet at the expense of α-helix detected for the pure SFD product could be completely avoided by the addition of polyols. In fact, helical content was even elevated by 0.4% (sucrose) - 0.8% (trehalose), while intermolecular β-sheet was reduced by 0.2% - 0.3%, respectively. Differences to the pure SFD particles must be considered significant, as standard deviations for intermolecular β-sheet determined in chapter 5.4.1 lay only between 0.3% and 0.4%. The small improvements over the untreated sample seem to be reliable as well.

Table 8.2: Changes to a-CT secondary structure after SFD using polyols as excipients.

Formulation	α-Helix	Intramol. β-sheet	Intermol. β-sheet
a-CT pure 100 mg/mL	-0.6%	+0.6%	+0.7%
+Sucrose 200 mg/mL	+0.8%	-0.2%	-0.3%
+Trehalose 200 mg/mL	+0.4%	-0.1%	-0.2%

Finally, overall enzyme stability of the protein/sugar formulations also exhibited superior results in comparison to the pure SFD product. Residual activity increased from 82.7% (SFD pure) to 85.5% (sucrose) and 95.3% (trehalose) (Fig. 8.2c). These findings were in agreement with the stabilizing effects to protein secondary and tertiary structure.Hence, it seems obvious that damage to a-CT during SFD at conservative settings (60 kHz ultrasonic nozzle at 3W) is mainly caused by the removal of water during the freeze-drying step. Additionally, trehalose exhibited superior stabilizing capacity than sucrose at the investigated concentrations.

SEM pictures of the a-CT/sucrose and a-CT/trehalose particles are shown in Fig. 8.3a+b, respectively. It is noticeable that porosity was greatly reduced in comparison to the pure 100 mg/mL SFD products. The sucrose particles exhibited a partially wrinkled, but mostly flat surface, while the combination with trehalose resulted in a completely smooth morphology. Rochelle et al. [2007] explained the wrinkled surface of TMD particles produced by SFD with a partial collapse of the freeze concentrate during the freeze-drying step. As trehalose exhibits an elevated T_g' in comparison to sucrose (- 27°C vs. – 31°C) [Meister et al. 2008], this could be the case as well for the sucrose particles. However, the very slow ramping step into secondary drying could still preserve most of the originally flat particle surface in the final powder. Furthermore, a particle that has been broken in half – visible in Fig. 8.3a – indicates that the spheres were not hollow in the inside which should improve their feasibility for e.g. transdermal powder delivery.

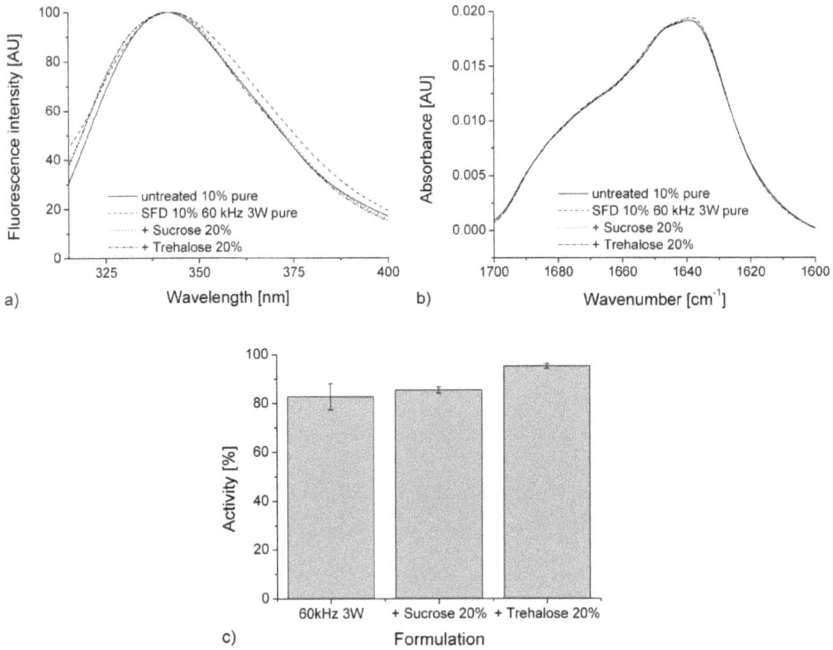

Fig. 8.2: SFD stabilizing experiments of a 100 mg/mL a-CT solution with help of sucrose and trehalose: a) Fluorescence spectra, b) FTIR amide I bands, c) Enzyme activity assay.

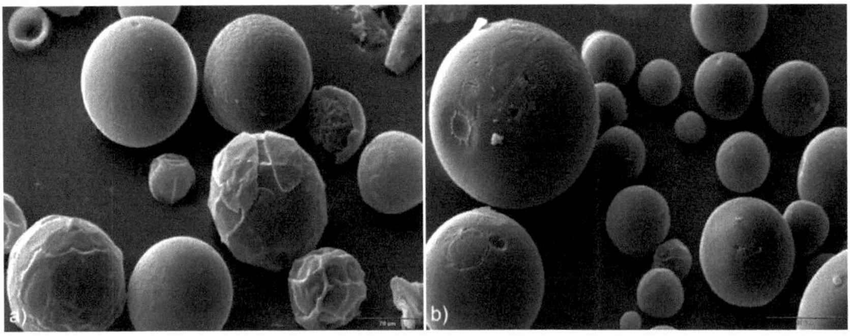

Fig. 8.3: SFD particles from 100 mg/mL a-CT solution using a) 200 mg/mL sucrose or b) 200 mg/mL trehalose as excipients (both 500x magnification).

8.1.3 Stabilization with complex formulations

Instead of using only one stabilizing excipient, more complex formulations have been applied in the past as well [Maa et al. 2004; Ziegler 2006; Rochelle et al. 2007]. The idea behind those more complex compositions was to combine multiple beneficial effects or at least to compensate for disadvantages of individual components. Trehalose, for example, generally exhibits a high hygroscopicity which is further augmented by the massive increase in surface area during SFD [Sonner 2002]. The addition of mannitol to the formulation has been used to reduce water uptake and increase particle rigidity [Maa et al. 2004]. Finally, dextran can be added to further enhance protein stability in the drying step by raising the T_g' of the formulation.

The resulting TMD formulations are completely amorphous immediately after the SFD process [Rochelle 2005]. This can cause protein instability in the final product as amorphous mannitol tends to recrystallize during long-term storage [Costantino et al. 1998]. As dextran exhibits an immunogenic potential [Hedin et al. 1982], it can be replaced by hydroxyethyl starch which offers similar stabilizing properties without the danger of anaphylactic reactions after parenteral application. On the downside, hydroxyethyl starch itself can cause severe local irritations at the injection site. a-CT was dissolved in the following 200 mg/mL excipient formulations: trehalose and hydroxyethyl starch at a ratio of 6:4 (TH 64); trehalose, mannitol and hydroxyethyl starch at a ratio of 3:3:4 (TMH 334), and trehalose, mannitol and dextran (MW=10 kDa) at a ratio of 3:3:4 (TMD 334).

The shift of the fluorescence maximum to 344.1 nm after SFD without excipients was greatly reduced using any of the combinations described above. TH 64 showed the lowest stabilizing capabilities resulting in a bathochrome shift to 343.0 nm which is still superior to the pure SFD results. Furthermore, TMD 334 and TMH 334 showed λ_{max} wavelengths of 342.2 nm and 342.3 nm, respectively, which represented a slight hypsochrome shift in comparison even to the untreated protein (Fig. 8.4a). Therefore, it can be stated that a-CT tertiary structure was completely stabilized by the complex formulations during the conservative SFD setup.

The native secondary structure of a-CT was only altered to a small extent during spray-freeze-drying of the pure enzyme solution (α-helix -0.6%, intramolecular β-sheet +0.6%, intermolecular β-sheet +0.7%). Therefore, no extensive improvements to secondary structure could be expected by the addition of excipients. Still, TH 64, TMD 334 and TMH 334 led to complete preservation of the native structures (Fig. 8.4b). In comparison to the amide I band of the untreated protein, intermolecular β-sheet was even slightly reduced (-0.3%), while α-helix increased by 0.5% at the most (especially for the TMH 334 formulation). No changes could be determined for intramolecular β-sheet (Table 8.3). Although these findings were detected for both TMD 334 and TMH 334 formulations, improvements detected over the untreated sample must be taken with caution as alterations in secondary structure lay mostly within the margin of error determined in chapter 5.4.1.

Table 8.3: The effect of complex formulations on the secondary structure of a-CT during SFD.

Formulation	α-Helix	Intramol. β-sheet	Intermol. β-sheet
a-CT pure 100 mg/mL	-0.6%	+0.6%	+0.7%
+TH 64 200 mg/mL	±0.0%	-0.3%	+0.3%
+TMH 334 200 mg/mL	+0.5%	+0.1%	-0.3%
+TMD 334 200 mg/mL	±0.0%	±0.0%	-0.1%

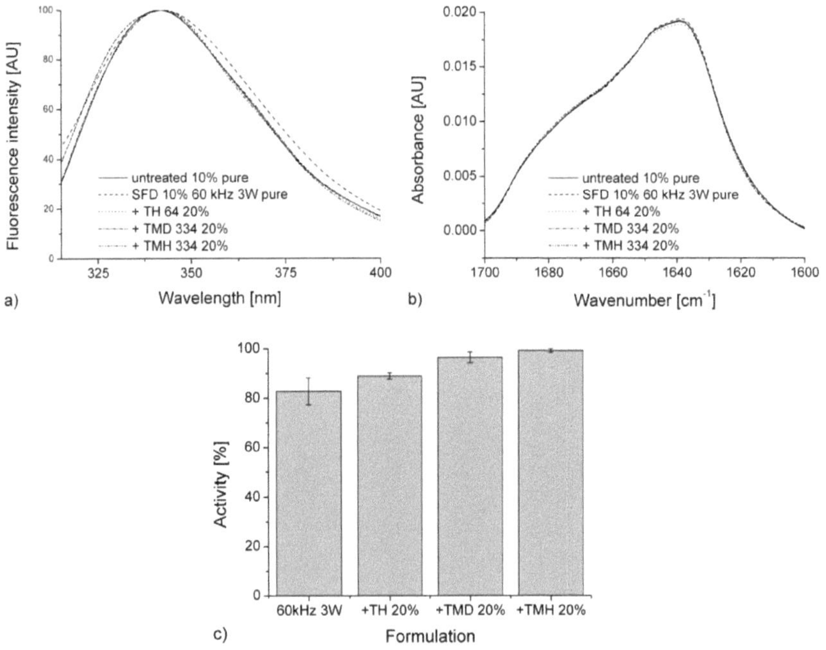

Fig. 8.4: Stabilization of 100 mg/mL a-CT particles using TH 64, TMD 334 and TMH 334 as excipient formulations: a) Fluorescence spectra, b) FTIR spectra, c) a-CT activity assay.

Evaluation of residual a-CT activity after SFD was in aggreement with the results determined for protein secondary and tertiary structure. Enzyme activity dropped to 82.7% after processing the pure enzyme solution, but could be increased by the addition of any of the three complex formulations. TH 64 was only able to elevate protein activity to 88.9% while TMD 334 and TMH 334 exhibited increases to 99.2% and 96.4%, respectively (Fig. 8.4c).

Fig. 8.5 shows SEM pictures of the manufactured SFD particles. Porosity was reduced in comparison to the pure 100 mg/mL a-CT solutions by using an overall solid content of 300 mg/mL (protein+excipients). Furthermore, no wrinkled surface, as could be seen in the sucrose particles in Fig. 8.3a, could be detected for any of the formulations although the combination TMD 334 is known to promote flow of the solid phase, leading to particle shrinkage [Maa et al. 2004]. Again, the slow ramping step in secondary drying in combination with a conservative shelf temperature of -24°C during primary drying seemed to have supported the preservation of the particle surface of the investigated formulations.

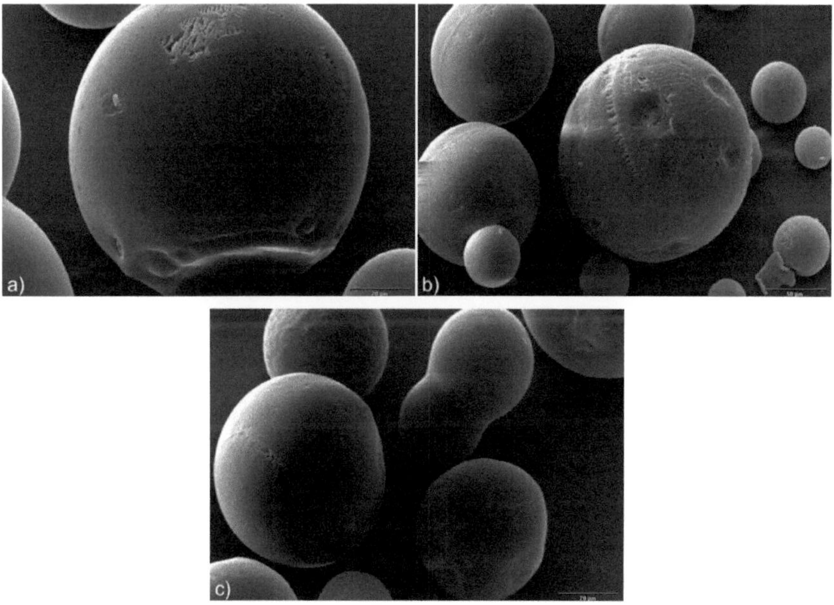

Fig. 8.5: SFD particles manufactured from 100 mg/mL a-CT solutions with a) TH 64 (1000x), b) TMD 334 (500x), c) TMH 334 (1000x).

8.1.4 Overall comparison and discussion

Under the conservative experimental setup (ultrasonic atomization at 60 kHz and 3W power input, followed by primary drying at -24°C shelf temperature), a-CT protein stability could almost be completely preserved by the incorporation of stabilizing excipients.

Maa et al. [2000] calculated the freezing time for a droplet with 10 µm diameter subjected to liquid nitrogen to be less than one millisecond. This causes the generation of many, very small ice crystals and thus, an extremely large surface area after the removal of ice by lyophilization. However, no clear trend between surface area and protein aggregation could be determined in their series of experiments. By adding 0.05% polysorbat 20, the aggregate content decreased slightly, but was still high. Therefore, they postulated that freezing stress could be the main reason for protein denaturation: if the ice front advances faster than a certain critical rate during freezing, it might alter protein conformation and lead to aggregation upon drying. In this work, addition of polysorbat 80 was not able to increase overall enzyme stability. Therefore, aggregation during atomization did not appear to be responsible for damage to α-chymotrypsin during SFD at the given droplet sizes. This is in agreement with the observation by Maa et al. [2000] and the results determined in chapter 6.4 where no correlation between droplet size (and thus air-liquid interface) and protein denaturation could be detected.

The protein solution containing trehalose exhibited superior stabilizing capabilities compared to the sucrose formulation. The exceptional stabilizing effect of trehalose and its mechanism of action have been reported previously in literature [Kaushik et al. 2003] and were confirmed by the results in this thesis. Enzyme stability could be completely preserved for at least short term storage if trehalose was used in combination with mannitol and either dextran or hydroxyethyl starch. However, this formulation could give rise to new stability problems as the completely amorphous mannitol tends to recrystallize during long-term storage (see chapter 8.1.3).

Analysis of the secondary and tertiary structure after the addition of excipients indicated that protein stabilization by preferential exclusion could be observed by FTIR and fluorescence spectroscopy. Even after the complete SFD process, intrinsic tryptophan fluorescence still exhibited a slight blueshift in comparison to the untreated protein. At the same time, intermolecular β-sheet content was reduced by values up to 0.3% while α-helix increased noticeably indicating an increase in native protein folding. As postulated by the preferential exclusion theory, a large protein-water interface would be thermodynamically unfavorable [Arakawa et al. 1991]. Higher protein folding, as encountered in the native state, reduces the available protein-water interface. It seems reasonable that this also leads to a relocation of the tryptophan residues towards the inside of the protein as well as to a decrease in intermolecular protein-protein interactions. Both effects have been determined by FTIR and fluorescence spectroscopy in this work.

In summary, damage to α-chymotrypsin could be connected to the stress experienced especially during the freeze-drying step. The addition of sugars helped preserving protein stability most likely by replacing the missing hydrogen bonds to the water molecules.

8.2 a-CT microparticles from high concentrated solutions (100 mg/mL): aggressive setup - 120 kHz 9W

8.2.1 Stabilization with sugars

As for the experiments performed with the conservative setup, sugars were added to the a-CT formulation, and stabilizing effects were investigated for an aggressive SFD setup (120 kHz, 9W). If freezing and water removal were again responsible for protein denaturation under the aggressive experimental setup, damage to a-CT should at least be partially avoided by the addition of sucrose or trehalose.

Using the 120 kHz nozzle at 9W for SFD without any excipients resulted in obvious damage to a-CT. The enzyme showed noticeable precipitation during reconstitution, and the solution had to be centrifuged prior to further analysis. λ_{max} of the fluorescence emission shifted to higher wavelengths from 342.2 nm to 345.5 nm, indicating disturbances to protein tertiary structure. Native α-helix and β-sheet content dropped by 3.2% and 2.9%, respectively. At the same time, intermolecular β-sheet increased by 4.2% which indicated the formation of protein aggregates. Extensive damage to overall a-CT stability could also be observed by enzyme activity assay which dropped to 32.2% after SFD (Fig. 8.6a-c).

As for the pure SFD particles, obvious precipitation was detectable during reconstitution of both formulations containing sugars, indicating the formation of insoluble aggregates. The bathochrome shift detected for the spray-freeze-dried pure a-CT solution could not be averted by the addition of sugars (Fig. 8.6a). Fluorescence maxima were in fact promoted to even higher wavelengths, resulting in λ_{max} values of 346.4 nm for sucrose and 346.3 nm for trehalose. These results indicated elevated damage to protein tertiary structure in spite of the added excipients, which was unexpected.

Analysis by FTIR spectroscopy revealed even stronger detrimental effects on the secondary structure of a-CT. Pure protein SFD particles already experienced substantial damage after the aggressive SFD process. The addition of the sucrose and trehalose, however, led to a further reduction of native structures (Fig. 8.6b). Intermolecular β-sheets were increased by values up to 8.2%, while native α-helix and intramolecular β-sheet contents were strongly reduced (see Table 8.4). This indicated massive damage to a-CT secondary structure during the SFD process.

Results from UV spectrometric assay also indicated slightly elevated damage to overall protein stability after the addition of excipients. While pure SFD particles still exhibited a residual activity of 32.2%, the incorporation of sucrose and trehalose led to a reduction in activity down to 22.5% and 30.8%, respectively (Fig. 8.6c).

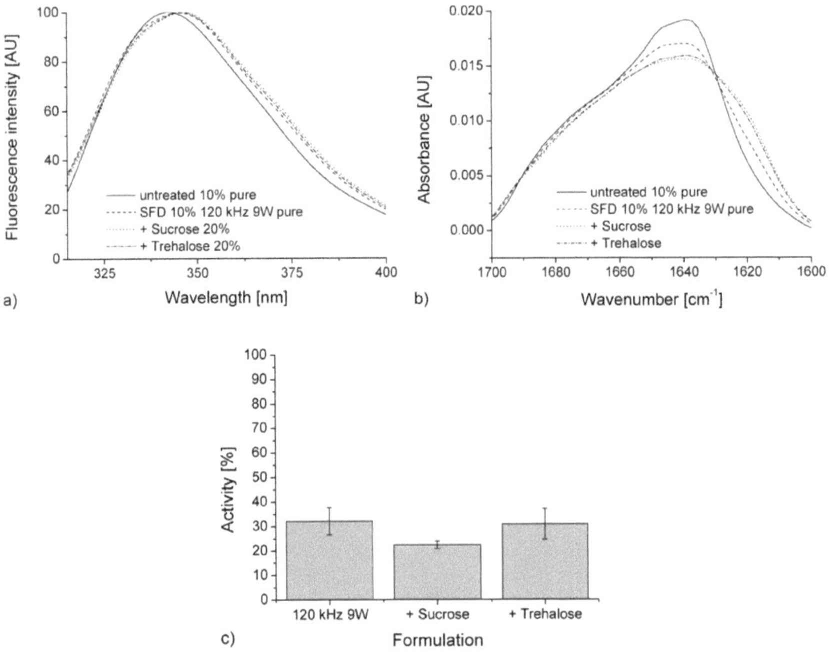

Fig. 8.6: Stability of 100 mg/mL a-CT solutions after SFD using aggressive atomization conditions: a) Fluorescence spectra, b) FTIR amide I bands, c) Enzyme activity assay.

Table 8.4: Effect of sucrose and trehalose on a-CT secondary structure after SFD.

Formulation	α-Helix	Intramol. β-sheet	Intermol. β-sheet
a-CT pure 100 mg/mL	-3.2%	-2.9%	+4.2%
+Sucrose 200 mg/mL	-6.8%	-3.1%	+8.2%
+Trehalose 200 mg/mL	-6.6%	-2.3%	+7.4%

In conclusion, results for the chymotrypsin solutions containing sugars were distributed roughly around or slightly below the same numbers as for the pure enzyme solution. Thus, the addition of sugars seemed to have had either negative effects or no effect at all on a-CT stability. Instead of rapid freezing or water removal, cavitation or temperature effects could be responsible for protein denaturation during the aggressive SFD setup.

Fig. 8.7 shows SEM pictures of the SFD particles generated under the aggressive experimental setup. No substantial differences between atomization using the 60 kHz nozzle at 3W and the 120 kHz nozzle at 9W were visible, except for the particle size. In both cases distinct, spherical particles were generated. The pure protein solution again exhibited a much more porous surface than the protein/excipients formulation due to its lower total solid content. However, the perfect spherical shape of some particles generated from preparations containing sugars was lost, possibly due to fusion between droplets during the atomization step. As no deformations were detected for the same formulations under the conservative setup, it might be possible that the occurrence of cavitation led to partially distorted droplet and particle shapes.

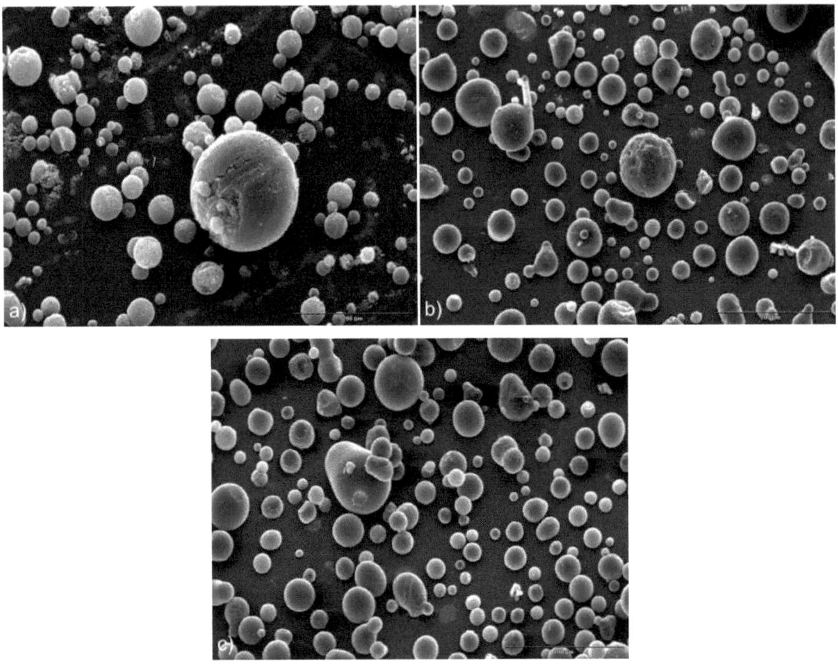

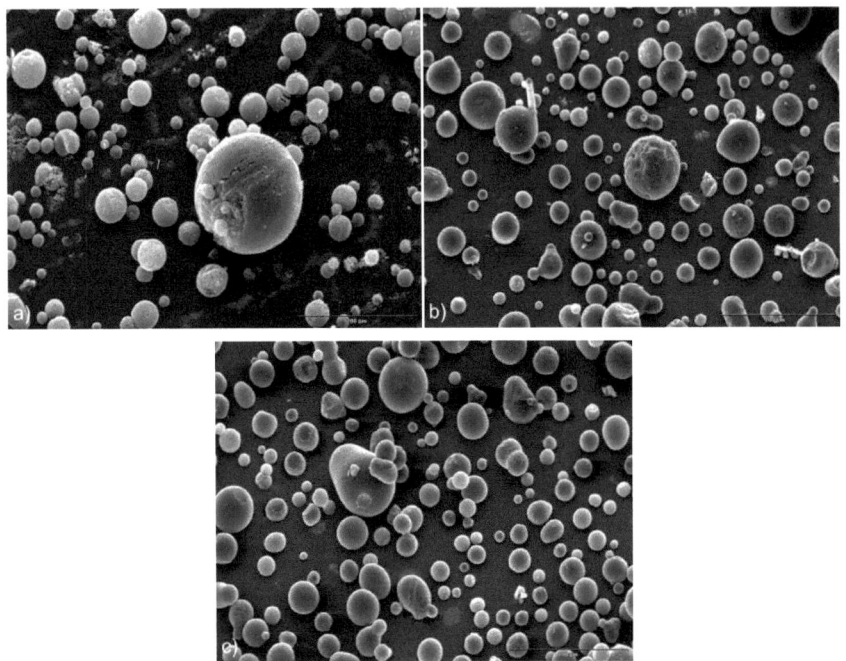

Fig. 8.7: SEM pictures of SFD particles generated from a) pure 100 mg/mL a-CT solution, b) 100 mg/mL a-CT+200 mg/mL sucrose solution, c) 100 mg/mL a-CT+200 mg/mL trehalose solution (all 200x magnification).

8.2.2 Stabilization with complex formulations

The same 200 mg/mL complex a-CT formulations that were used in the conservative setup (TH 64, TMD 334, TMH 334) were then evaluated using the 120 kHz nozzle at 9W for atomization. During reconstitution massive precipitation was once more visible for all three formulations investigated, making it necessary to centrifuge the samples prior to further analysis.

Fluorescence maxima were shifted to wavelengths between 345.1 nm (TH 64) and 345.7 nm (TMH 334) which presented minimal improvements over the sugar formulations discussed in the previous chapter (Fig. 8.8a). However, no stabilization of protein tertiary structure was accomplished as λ_{max} of the pure SFD product already laid at 345.5 nm.

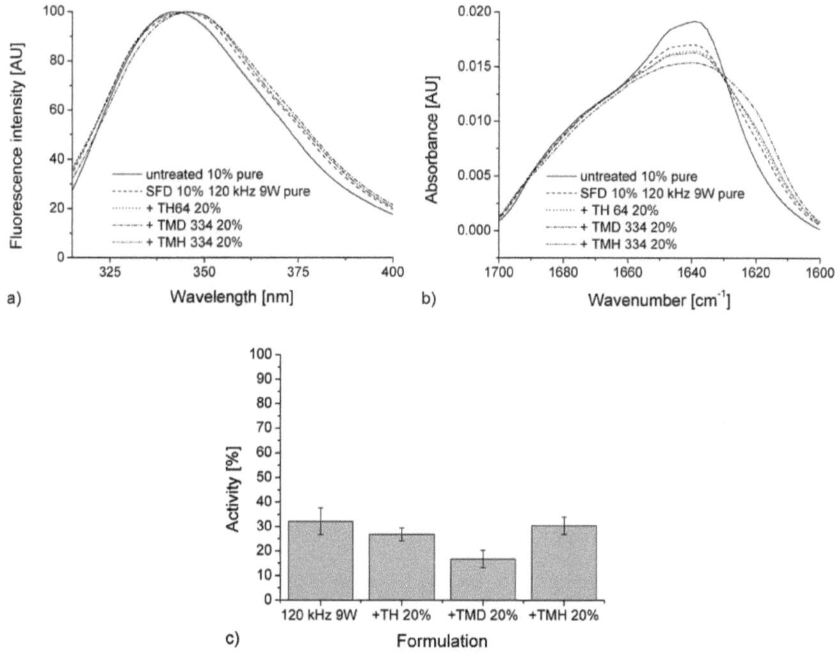

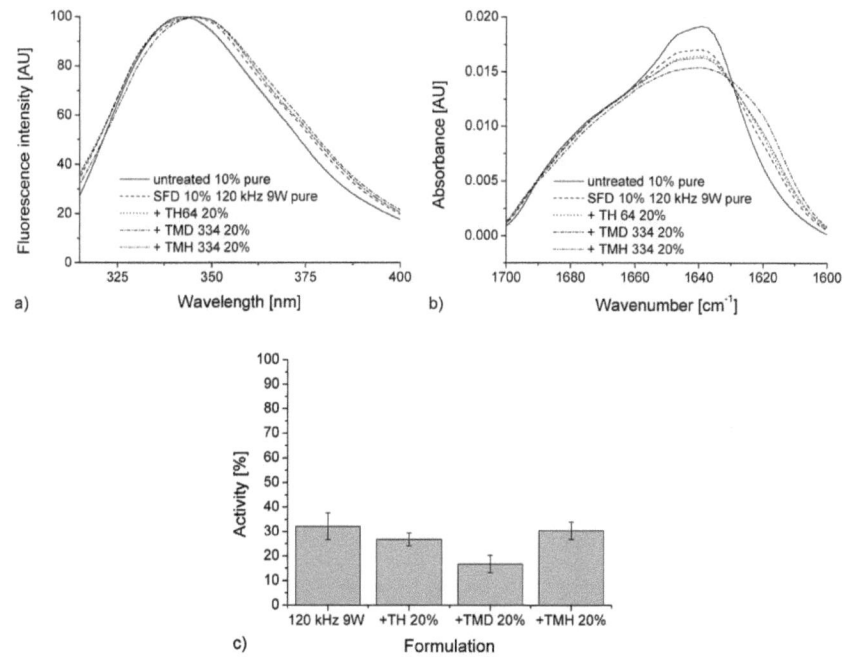

Fig. 8.8: Stabilization experiments for the aggressive SFD setup using complex formulations of classical excipients: a) Fluorescence spectra, b) FTIR amide I bands, c) a-CT activity assay.

The secondary structure of a-CT was even stronger damaged than its tertiary structure, just like determined earlier for the simple sugar formulations. Highest protein denaturation was observed using the TMD 334 combination as additive. α-Helix experienced a severe drop by 7.3% while the loss of intramolecular β-sheet was less pronounced (-3.2%). Additionally, intermolecular β-sheet increased substantially by 8.5%, which can be linked to extreme damage to protein secondary structure (Fig. 8.8b). As can be seen in Table 8.5, utilization of TH 64 and TMH 334 resulted in only slightly lower levels of damage than the TMD 334 formulation when used under aggressive settings.

Damage to a-CT tertiary and secondary structure could also be linked to overall protein stability. In comparison to the SFD experiment using the pure enzyme solution, the formulations containing excipients showed similar or even inferior stability (Fig. 8.8c). Highest activity was achieved for the a-CT/TMH 334 formulation (30.4%) which is still slightly below the activity of the pure SFD particles (32.2%). Results for the TH 64 (26.8%) and TMD 334 (16.8%) formulations were even worse.

Table 8.5: SFD experiments with complex a-CT formulations under aggressive conditions

Formulation	α-Helix	Intramol. β-sheet	Intermol. β-sheet
a-CT pure 100 mg/mL	-3.2%	-2.9%	+4.2%
+TH 64 200 mg/mL	-4.7%	-1.9%	+5.1%
+TMH 334 200 mg/mL	-4.8%	-3.0%	+5.9%
+TMD 334 200 mg/mL	-7.3%	-3.2%	+8.5%

As can be seen in Fig. 8.9, the final particles did not differ from the other formulated SFD products. The individual spheres were partially merged which led to elongated particles that lost their perfect round shape. As no collapse or shrinkage of the particles was visible, the deformations seemed to have taken place during the spraying step rather than the subsequent freeze-drying run.

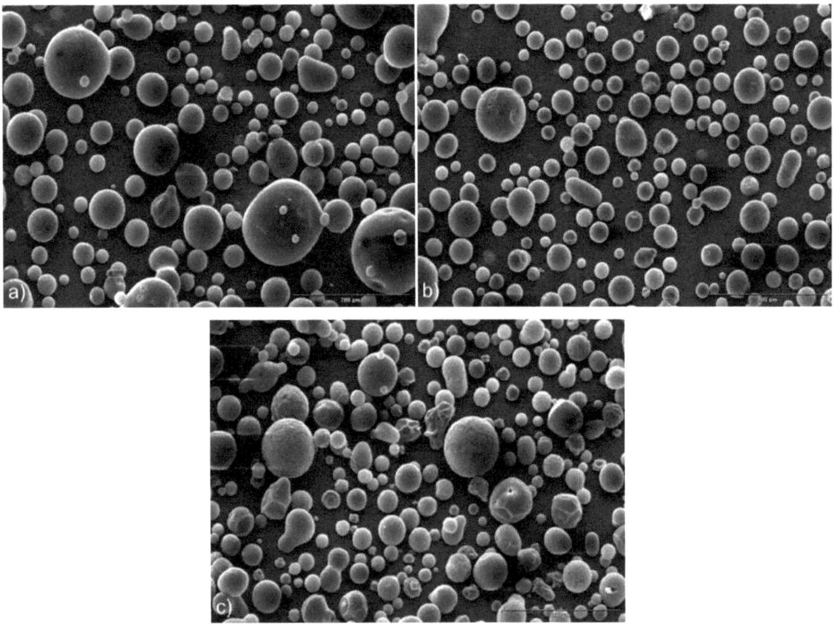

Fig. 8.9: SEM pictures of SFD particles from high concentrated a-CT formulations using a) TH 64, b) TMD 334 and c) TMH 334 as excipients (all 200x magnification).

8.2.3 Ascorbic acid

As stabilization could not be achieved by application of classic lyo- and cryoprotectants, the addition of ascorbic acid as an antioxidant excipient was evaluated. Based on the results presented in chapters 7.4 and 7.5, temperature effects and free radicals generated through cavitation could both be responsible for the high protein damage under aggressive experimental conditions. However, strong damage due to the nozzle's heat dissipation seemed unlikely considering the temperature-time-profile of the 120 kHz nozzle at 9W: Temperature increased comparably fast within the first few minutes, but as the volume of SFD solutions usually did not exceed 2 mL, the whole atomization step was finished within two minutes at the usual liquid feed rate. Thus, only the latter part of the 2 mL formulation would have been subjected to temperature stress of 65°C at most, which could not explain the severe level of damage observed in the experiments above. By adding ascorbic acid at molar ratio of 1:2 (protein:excipient) protein damage should at least be reduced if oxidation by free radicals played a key role during SFD at 120 kHz, 9W.

Noticeable precipitation occurred during redissolving of the formulation, indicating that substantial protein damage was induced in spite of the incorporation of ascorbic acid. Before analysis, samples had to be centrifuged to remove any insoluble aggregates.

In Fig. 8.10a, the fluorescence spectra of the untreated and the spray-freeze-dried a-CT solutions with and without ascorbic acid are shown. λ_{max} was still noticeably shifted (+2.0 nm) to higher wavelengths, but to a lesser extent than the pure a-CT particles after reconstitution (+3.1 nm). Hence, tertiary structure underwent fewer perturbations in the presence of ascorbic acid even though no complete stabilization could be achieved.

a-CT secondary structure could also be stabilized to a certain extent by the addition of an antioxidant (Fig. 8.10b). Quantification by the PLS algorithm showed that protein damage was significantly reduced in comparison to the pure SFD experiment (Table 8.6). However, results still indicated no complete preservation of protein secondary structure. α-Helix and intramolecular β-sheet were reduced by 2.0% and 0.9%, respectively, while intermolecular β-sheet increased by 2.0%.

As the protein's secondary and tertiary structure have often been linked to its residual activity in previous experiments, it is not surprising that a-CT activity was improved as well by the addition of ascorbic acid. While the pure a-CT particles performed at 32.2% activity, 69.9% of the residual activity could be preserved with the antioxidant. This was quite impressive considering the residual activities determined for the previous formulations.

Table 8.6: Stabilization of a-CT during aggressive atomization settings with help of ascorbic acid.

Formulation	α-Helix	Intramol. β-sheet	Intermol. β-sheet
a-CT pure 100 mg/mL	-3.2%	-2.9%	+4.2%
+Ascorb. acid	-2.0%	-0.9%	+2.0%

The morphology of the final product consisted once again of highly porous, spherical particles typical for SFD at an intermediate solid content (Fig. 8.10c). Partial merging of the particles could be observed just like determined in the previous experiments using the aggressive atomization step. Ascorbic acid was applied at a very low concentration and thus is not visible in the final product

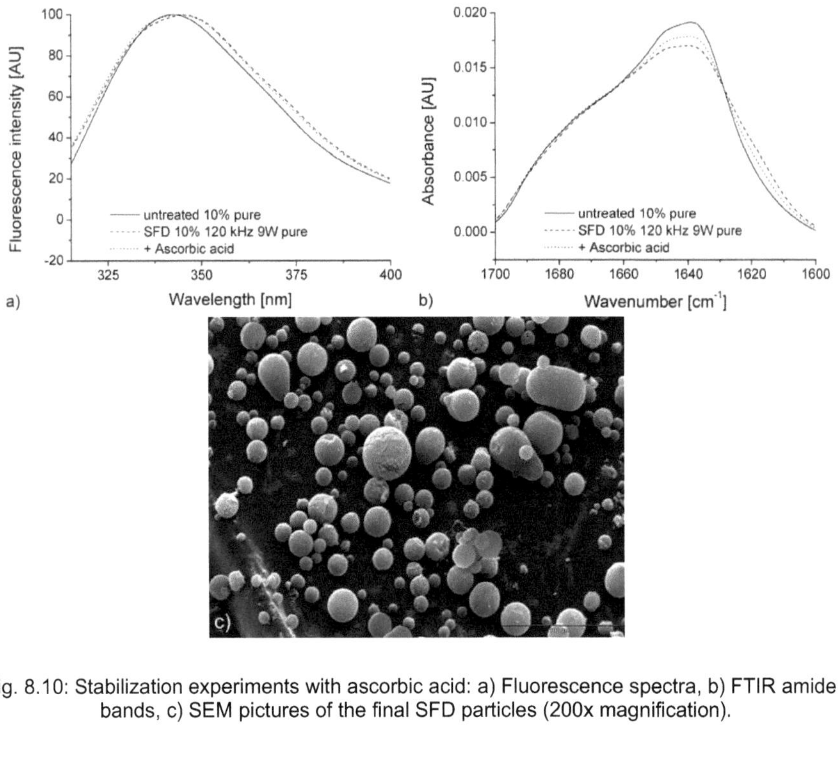

Fig. 8.10: Stabilization experiments with ascorbic acid: a) Fluorescence spectra, b) FTIR amide I bands, c) SEM pictures of the final SFD particles (200x magnification).

8.2.4 Overall comparison and discussion

From the formulation experiments performed using the 120 kHz nozzle at 9W the following conclusion can be deducted:

First, atomization seemed to be the critical processing step for a-CT during SFD at rather aggressive conditions. The pure 100 mg/mL a-CT solution suffered elevated damage in regard to secondary and tertiary structures as well as enzyme activity if atomization was performed at 9W using the 120 kHz nozzle during SFD. As increases in power input do not change the droplet size distribution towards lower diameters (as long as homogeneous atomization is still provided) [Sono-Tek 2009], higher protein damage cannot be explained by changes in surface area and elevated protein/interface adsorption.

Second, neither sugars alone nor more complex formulations were able to stabilize a-CT during SFD at 120 kHz, 9W. Performance of the solutions containing stabilizers was equivalent to or even slightly below pure spray-freeze-dried a-CT. This is somewhat surprising, because at least minimal improvements should have been noticeable by the addition of lyo- and cryoprotectants, according to preferential exclusion and water replacement theories [Allison et al. 1998]. Possible reasons for the inferior performance of these formulations are discussed in the following paragraph. However, improvements in overall stability could be detected by adding ascorbic acid as excipient to the pure enzyme solution. Hence, it seems obvious that stabilization occurred by preventing oxidation of the enzyme. This strongly suggests that the prevention of cavitation presents the key mechanism in stabilization of a-CT under aggressive atomization conditions.

There are three possible reasons for the surprisingly bad results determined for the classic SFD formulations: First, stabilization by cryoprotectants could have been lost due to phase separation during freezing [Maa et al. 2000]. However, X-ray diffraction analysis of freshly prepared a-CT/TMD 334 particles showed a completely amorphous product [Vonhoff 2007]. Therefore, no phase separation was assumed that could possibly explain protein denaturation. Second, the stabilizing influence of the excipients could have been overcompensated by detrimental effects generated during the aggressive atomization step. As stated in chapter 7.5.3, cavitation is dependent on numerous factors. Increasing the solid content of the solution threefold (from 100 mg/mL pure a-CT to 300 mg/mL after adding the excipients) affects several factors at once, such as viscosity, density or surface tension. Therefore, it is very likely that the high-concentrated formulations exhibited different behavior during the atomization step than the pure enzyme solution. However, no evidence of augmented cavitation under these conditions could be found, making it difficult to verify this theory. Alternatively, no stabilization could have been achieved at all by the addition of excipients. This would be the case if the protein structure had already been damaged in a way that made stabilization by cryo- and lyoprotectants impossible (e.g. oxidation, disulfide bond breakage, etc.). Therefore, differences between formulations containing classic stabilizer would only reflect the varying atomization conditions under aggressive atomization settings. This would mean that actual differences between the pure SFD product and the formulated enzyme were rather small, but the spraying stress varied considerably due to the occurrence of elevated temperatures and high cavitation effects. Additionally, the inhomogeneity in liquid feed rate (see chapter 7.2) could have reduced the reproducibility of the atomization step even further. This would be in agreement with the high standard deviations seen during the cavitation experiments for the 120 kHz nozzle at 9W (chapter 7.5). Possible outliers in chapter 6.4 and fluctuations detected in the temperature-time-profiles at demanding settings could fit into this theory as well. Additionally, most of the results gained from the formulation experiments were pretty close to the pure SFD particles, except for the FTIR analyses which revealed noticeably higher damage.

The exact reason for the inadequate performance of the formulated solutions could not be determined by the experimental design used in this thesis, but should definitely be considered in future works.

9. Conclusions

This thesis deals with the preparation of protein microparticles by spray-freeze-drying and the effects of the process on protein secondary and tertiary structure. SFD is a relatively new process for particle preparation, which consists of numerous unit operations and hence is still not thoroughly explored. In general, a liquid feed solution is atomized with a two-fluid or an ultrasound nozzle above a cryogen. The fine droplet spray is almost instantly frozen upon contact with the liquid and can be transferred onto the pre-cooled shelves of a freeze-dryer after the majority of the cryogen has boiled off. The final powder is prepared by sublimation of the ice at low temperature and pressure. The properties of the final product are dependent, amongst others, on solution concentration, excipient formulation, atomization conditions, type of cryogen and the freeze-drying cycle. This leads to a vast number of possible combinations, making a comprehensive experimental design almost impossible. Therefore, lyophilization was performed under very conservative conditions in this thesis to minimize its influence on product properties. Additionally, only LN_2 was used as cryogen in this work, as it exhibits superior handling in contrast to e.g. liquid propane or isopentane and is not flammable.

The first part of this thesis covered the development of an FTIR method for the determination of protein secondary structure, which is directly linked to protein stability. FTIR spectroscopy offers a great amount of flexibility during sample recording, and therefore can provide valuable information about the SFD process. Prior to analyzing secondary structure during SFD, a new method of evaluation had to be established. Other previously desribed methods suffered from either reduced informational content (such as evaluation by correlation coefficient) or a high degree of subjectivity (e.g. evaluation by peak fitting), and were therefore considered inadequate for the needs of the research presented in this thesis. By applying an iPLS algorithm, shape and intensity of the area-normalized and baseline-corrected amide I bands of 16 different proteins were correlated to protein secondary structure. This made it possible to quantify protein denaturation by the transition of native structures (α-helix, intramolecular β-sheet) to intermolecular β-sheet. Only minimal pre-processing was necessary, which drastically reduced subjectivity by user input. Validity of the calibration standards was assured by comparing FTIR evaluations by peak fitting to data from X-ray analysis. Both techniques showed very good agreement for most of the proteins. Additionally, precision of the evaluation of denatured proteins had to be assessed. As no X-ray data was available for denatured proteins, results from the iPLS quantification procedure of HSA and glucagon were compared with peak fitting and CD. Very good correlation could be determined between iPLS and peak fitting. This was expected, as evaluations are based on the same amide I bands. Still, this outcome supports the credibility of the results determined by calibration curves. Comparison between iPLS and CD revealed minor deviations caused by the different operational setup of the two methods. However, both evaluations revealed that roughly 70% of native α-helix and β-sheet were transformed into intermolecular β-sheet during denaturation, thus supporting the quantification approach performed in this thesis. Finally, formation of aggregates could be linked to increasing intermolecular β-sheet content by including results from SEC-HPLC. Therefore, evaluation of protein secondary structure could also be employed for objectively assessing protein denaturation and aggregation during SFD. Precision of quantification could presumably be further increased by including denatured protein standards in the calibration step as well. Furthermore, it would be promising to evaluate the performance of the iPLS algorithm regarding solid samples. The amide I bands of both liquid and solid samples incorporate the same molecular vibrations and therefore, only little modifications should be necessary for transferring the algorithm. This would greatly increase its field of application.

The second part of this thesis investigated the influence of atomization conditions on protein secondary and tertiary structure as well as residual enzyme activity during SFD. a-CT and HSA, used as model proteins during those experiments, were chosen due to their differences in secondary structure. While the first one exhibits a structure consisting of predominantly β-sheet, the latter one is made up of mostly α-helix. The proteins were prepared without further excipients at both low and high concentrations and evaluated after the following processing steps:

- Atomization
- Atomization, freezing and thawing back at room temperature
- The complete spray-freeze-drying process.

Throughout the entire study, HSA exhibited extraordinary stability. Increasing the concentration form 10 mg/mL to 100 mg/mL led to only little changes in protein secondary and tertiary structures. Possible unfolding still could have occurred during lyophilization but was not detected in the reconstituted samples. Therefore, HSA proved to be suitable for the SFD process, irrespective of the applied atomization conditions and protein concentrations. Damage to a-CT, on the other hand, was dependent on the frequency of the ultrasonic nozzle during atomization. Highest stability was achieved for the 60 kHz nozzle, while the 25 kHz nozzle inflicted highest damage during each of the processing steps. The 48 kHz and 120 kHz setups positioned themselves in between the above mentioned results. Part of the damage during atomization could be averted by instant freezing after spraying into LN_2. However, subsequent water removal by lyophilization annihilated any positive effects of the freezing step and yielded even higher damage. Increasing the protein concentration from 10 mg/mL to 100 mg/mL further augmented the detrimental effects by SFD. As the nozzle frequency determines the resulting droplet size, one would suspect increasing protein damage with higher frequencies and increasing specific surface area. However, this was not the case. The 25 kHz nozzle, generating the largest droplets, inflicted highest protein damage. Therefore, other factors than adsorption of a-CT to the droplet/air interface appear to have been the driving force for protein instability.

Changes to protein secondary and tertiary structure were interrelated, but tertiary structure showed a slightly higher responsivity concerning protein denaturation. a-CT activity, showing the highest level of sensitivity, supported evaluations by FTIR and fluorescence spectroscopy. Generally, higher standard deviations were observed during all analyses if elevated protein damage was induced.

A thorough comparison of the individual ultrasound nozzles was performed in the third part of this thesis. In a first series of experiments, the influence of different pumps on the homogeneity of the liquid feed rate was evaluated. Under the given experimental setup no significant differences could be detected, irrespective of the applied conditions. The same was true for the influence of the different pumps on the resulting particle size distributions. Although, these results might be biased by the merge of droplets after atomization, the ultrasound nozzles delivered good spraying performance in spite of slight fluctuations in liquid feed homogeneity. Next, temperatures of the spray cloud in correlation to the nozzle frequency were investigated. Higher frequencies and atomization powers led to increased heat output, peaking at 80°C for the 120 kHz design. At more aggressive spraying conditions (e.g. 120 kHz, 9W), obvious fluctuations in the temperature-time-profile were detectable. As temperatures alone could not be responsible for elevated protein damage in chapter 6, the occurrence of ultrasonic cavitation was analyzed in a third series of experiments. Cavitation leads to the generation of free radicals that can oxidize proteins as well as added excipients. Three marker solutions were subjected to nozzle activity and then evaluated for their increase in fluorescence (TA) or absorbance (KI, Fe). While distribution of the results was still pretty narrow at 3W power input, noticeable differences were detectable at higher settings. The 60 kHz nozzle showed lowest cavitation effects, followed by the 48 kHz and the 120 kHz nozzles. The latter one induced very strong oxidation, almost comparable to an ultrasound homogenizer. The 25 kHz nozzle, however, could not be evaluated as no continuous operation was achievable under the experimental setup. This is especially disadvantageous as this nozzle type induced the highest protein damage during the experiments performed in chapter 6. Comparable to observations in other experiments at aggressive atomization conditions, standard deviations increased substantially at 9W power input, indicating inhomogeneity during spraying.

In the fourth and last part of this thesis, different formulations containing a mixture of a-CT and excipients were evaluated for their stability. HSA was excluded from these experiments, as it was not noticeably affected during the previous SFD experiments. a-CT was processed at different conditions: At 60 kHz and 3W, the enzyme could be stabilized almost completely by the addition of trehalose or a mixture of TMD or TMH. Polysorbat 80 was not able to noticeably prevent protein damage which indicated that adsorption to the air/liquid interface only played a subordinate role during the SFD experiments performed in this thesis. Therefore, damage to a-CT under conservative atomization conditions seemed to be mostly caused by the freezing and drying steps, as it is the case during conventional freeze-drying. Under aggressive atomization conditions (120 kHz, 9W), a-CT could not be stabilized anymore with these classic excipients. Evaluation of secondary and tertiary structure as well as enzyme activity consistently showed comparable or even inferior protein stability. Hence, other factors than the freezing and drying stress must be taken into account. By adding ascorbic acid as an antioxidant, enzyme stability could be preserved to a certain extent. This strongly indicated that oxidation due to cavitation effects played a key role in protein damage at aggressive conditions. Sugars and polymers mostly preserve the native conformation of a protein during the freezing and drying step. Hence, cavitation could also explain the inferior stabilizing capability of those excipients when atomization was performed at 120 kHz and 9W.

In summary, SFD has shown to be capable of generating microparticles with a high protein load. No general assumptions concerning protein stability can be made, as a-CT and HSA performed very differently during the individual processing steps. When atomized at conservative conditions, the additional stress factors posed by the atomization step did not noticeably affect protein stability. This means that proteins could readily be stabilized by the addition of classic cryo- and lyoprotectants. The investigated ultrasonic nozzles were not necessarily superior to their two-fluid counterparts in regard to protein stability. More aggressive atomization conditions increased the influence of cavitation stress, thereby potentially destabilizing the protein. On the other hand, ultrasound nozzles offer the possibility to spray small volumes with low liquid flow rates. In addition, reduced agitation of LN_2 noticeably improved feasibility of the SFD process.

By creating an iPLS quantification algorithm for FTIR spectroscopy, investigation of protein secondary structure could be incorporated as an objective and fast standard evaluation method. Even though sensitivity was lower than e.g. enzyme activity assay, it proved to deliver precise information on protein structure and stability. The adoption of the algorithm towards solid samples would make it possible to investigate spray-freeze-drying during the individual processing steps separately. In regard to cavitation analysis, a refined experimental design would be valuable that is capable of measuring the in-situ generation of free radicals from a standard SFD setup. This would allow data collection from a more representative point of view. Additionally, an experimental setup capable of evaluating the 25 kHz nozzle design could provide further insight into atomization stress. Investigation of the fluctuations in temperature and oxidative stress, especially at demanding process conditions, could be another starting point for enhancing the understanding of possible stress factors during spray-freeze-drying. Finally, evaluation of the stabilizing potential of other antioxidants or combinations of antioxidants with classic excipients seems promising. These formulations could deliver highest benefit as protein damage during SFD is most likely caused by both chemical and physical instabilities at aggressive conditions. All of the above described advancements could further increase insight into this rather complicated manufacturing technology during future works.

10. Zusammenfassung

Diese Dissertation behandelt die Herstellung von Mikropartikeln durch Sprühgefriertrocknung und deren Einfluss auf die Sekundär- und Tertiärstruktur von Proteinen. SFD ist ein relativ neuartiges Herstellungsverfahren für Partikel, das durch eine Vielzahl an Variablen beeinflusst wird. Vermutlich konnte die Sprühgefriertrocknung auch aus diesem Grunde bis heute nicht umfassend untersucht werden. Das Funktionsprinzip beruht auf der Zerstäubung einer Lösung mittels Zweistoff- oder Ultraschalldüse über einem flüssigen Kühlmittel. Die feinen Tröpfchen gefrieren fast augenblicklich bei Kontakt mit der Flüssigkeit und werden nach Verdampfen des Kühlmittels auf die vorgekühlten Stellflächen eines Gefriertrockners überführt. Dort wird das Eis bei geringem Druck und niedrigen Temperaturen sublimiert, wodurch das fertige Endprodukt erhalten wird. Die Eigenschaften des Endprodukts hängen unter anderem von der Konzentration der Lösung, der Zusammensetzung der Hilfsstoffformulierung, den Zerstäubungsbedingungen, sowie der Art des Kühlmittels und dem Gefriertrocknungszyklus ab. Dieses führt zu einer enormen Anzahl an Kombinationsmöglichkeiten, was es nahezu unmöglich macht alle Bedingungen in einem Versuchsdesign zu berücksichtigen. Deshalb wurde in der vorliegenden Arbeit ein konservativer Gefriertrocknungszyklus gewählt, um dessen Einfluss auf die Eigenschaften des Endprodukts zu minimieren. Zudem wurde ausschließlich flüssiger Stickstoff als Kühlmittel genutzt, da dieser eine einfache Handhabung ohne jede Explosionsgefahr aufweist.

Der erste Teil dieser Arbeit beschreibt die Entwicklung einer FTIR-Methode zur Quantifizierung der Sekundärstruktur von Proteinen, welche in direktem Zusammenhang zur Stabilität eines Proteins steht. Darüber hinaus zeichnet sich FTIR-Spektroskopie durch vielfältige Möglichkeiten für die Vermessung von Proben aus und kann deshalb wertvolle Informationen sowohl aus Zwischen- als auch den Endprodukten des SFD Prozesses liefern. Bevor es jedoch möglich war die Sekundärstruktur während der Sprühgefriertrocknung zu analysieren, musste zunächst eine neue Auswertungsmethode entwickelt werden. Früher veröffentlichte Auswertungen litten entweder an einem niedrigen Informationsgehalt (z.B. die Auswertung per Korrelationskoeffizient) oder an einem hohen Grad an Subjektivität (z.B. „peak fitting"). Aus diesem Grunde waren diese Methoden inadäquat für die Ansprüche dieser Dissertation.

Mittels eines iPLS Algorithmus wurden Form und Intensität der flächennormierten und baselinekorrigierten Amid-I-Banden von 16 verschiedenen Proteinen mit den wichtigsten

Sekundärstrukturen korreliert. So wurde es möglich, die Denaturierung eines Proteins aufgrund des Übergangs von nativen Strukturen (α-helix, intramolekulares β-Faltblatt) hin zu intermolekularem β-Faltblatt zu quantifizieren. Dabei war nur eine minimale Vorbearbeitung der Daten nötig, was subjektive Einflüsse seitens des Benutzers stark reduzierte bis komplett eliminierte. Die Richtigkeit der Kalibrierungsstandards wurde überprüft, indem Ergebnisse von peak fitting mit Daten aus der Röntgenstrukturanalyse abgeglichen wurden. Beide Techniken zeigten für einen Großteil der Proteine eine sehr gute Übereinstimmung. Anschließend musste die Zuverlässigkeit der Quantifizierung bei denaturierten Proteinen bestimmt werden. Da dafür keine Röntgenstrukturen zur Verfügung standen, wurden Veränderungen der Sekundärstruktur von HSA und Glucagon (bestimmt mittels iPLS) mit Daten von peak fitting und CD verglichen. Zwischen iPLS und peak fitting wurde eine hervorragende Übereinstimmung festgestellt. Dies war zu erwarten, da beide Methoden auf den gleichen Amid-I-Banden beruhen. Dennoch unterstützt dieses Ergebnis die Glaubwürdigkeit der Ergebnisse, welche mittels Kalibriergeraden bestimmt wurden. Der Vergleich zwischen iPLS und CD offenbarte geringfügige Abweichungen, welche durch die grundlegend unterschiedlichen Funktionsprinzipien der beiden Methoden bedingt waren. Trotzdem zeigten beide Auswertungen, dass ca. 70% der nativen Helix und Faltblatt Strukturen von HSA während der Denaturierung in intermolekulares β-Faltblatt umgewandelt werden. Auch dies unterstützt den Auswertungsansatz, der in dieser Dissertation praktiziert wurde. Zuletzt konnte noch die Bildung von Aggregaten mit zunehmendem intermolekularem β-Faltblatt in Zusammenhang gebracht werden, indem die Ergebnisse einer Größenausschlusschromatographie mit einbezogen wurden. Mit diesem Verfahren kann die Bestimmung der Protein Sekundärstruktur benutzt werden, um objektiv Denaturierung und Aggregation während der Sprühgefriertrocknung zu quantifizieren. Die Präzision der Auswertung könnte vermutlich noch weiter verbessert werden, indem denaturierte Proteine als Standards mit in die Kalibrierung übernommen werden. Darüber hinaus erscheint es vielversprechend die Leistung des iPLS in Bezug auf feste Proben zu bestimmen. Die Amid-I-Bande von sowohl flüssigen als auch festen Proben wird von den gleichen Molekülvibrationen erzeugt. Demnach sollten bereits geringen Modifikationen genügen, um den Algorithmus auf Feststoffe zu übertragen, was dessen Anwendungsgebiet deutlich erweitern würde.

Im zweiten Teil dieser Dissertation wurde der Einfluss verschiedener Sprühbedingungen auf die Sekundär- und Tertiärstruktur sowie die verbleibende Enzymaktivität nach der Sprühgefriertrocknung untersucht. a-CT und HSA wurden aufgrund ihrer Unterschiede in der Sekundärstruktur als Modellproteine ausgewählt. Während ersteres eine ausgeprägte β-Faltblatt Struktur aufweist besteht das Zweite hauptsächlich aus α-Helix Ketten. Die Proteine wurden ohne jegliche Hilfsstoffe sowohl in niedriger als auch in hoher Konzentration gelöst und nach den folgenden Herstellungsschritten untersucht:

- Direkt nach dem Versprühen
- Nach Versprühen, Gefrieren und anschließendem Auftauen bei Raumtemperatur
- Nach dem gesamten SFD Prozess.

HSA zeigte eine außergewöhnliche Stabilität während der einzelnen Prozessschritte. Eine Erhöhung der Konzentration von 10 mg/mL auf 100 mg/mL führte nur zu geringfügigen Änderungen in der Sekundär- und Tertiärstruktur. Möglicherweise kam es während des Gefriertrocknens zu einer reversiblen Proteinentfaltung. Dies konnte aber durch die rekonstituierten Proben nicht belegt werden. Damit konnte gezeigt werden, dass HSA gut für die Sprühgefriertrocknung geeignet ist – unabhängig von Zerstäubungsbedingungen und Proteinkonzentrationen. Die Schädigung von a-CT war dagegen abhängig von der Zerstäubungsfrequenz der Düse. Die höchste Stabilität erzielte die 60 kHz Düse während die 25 kHz Düse den höchsten Schaden hervorrief. Die 48 kHz und 120 kHz Ausführungen positionierten sich zwischen den oben erwähnten Ergebnissen. Ein Teil des Schadens während des Zerstäubungsschritts konnte durch sofortiges Einfrieren in flüssigem Stickstoff vermieden werden. Die anschließende Entfernung von Wasser während des Gefriertrocknungsschritts machte jedoch jeglichen positiven Effekt des Einfrierens wieder zunichte und verursachte starke Schäden. Eine Erhöhung der Konzentration von 10 mg/mL auf 100 mg/mL verstärkte die Auswirkungen der jeweiligen Prozessschritte. Trotzdem folgten die Ergebnisse dem gleichen Trend wie bei den niedrig konzentrierten Ansätzen. Da die Düsenfrequenz durch die entstehende Tröpfchengröße bestimmt ist, sollten verstärkte nachteilige Auswirkungen mit zunehmender Frequenz und damit größerer spezifischen Oberfläche zu vermuten sein. Dies war jedoch nicht der Fall. Die 25 kHz Düse verursachte den höchsten Schaden obwohl sie die größten Tröpfchen produzierte. Insofern schienen noch andere Faktoren als die Adsorption von a-CT an die Grenzfläche zwischen Flüssigkeit und Gas für die Instabilität des Proteins verantwortlich zu sein.

Änderungen in der Sekundär- und Tertiärstruktur hingen direkt miteinander zusammen. Die Tertiärstruktur sprach jedoch etwas direkter auf Veränderungen durch Proteindenaturierung an. Die Auswertung der Enzym Aktivität zeigte im Allgemeinen die höchste Sensitivität und unterstützte die Ergebnisse von FTIR und Fluoreszenzspektroskopie. Generell nahm die Standardabweichung zu, wenn dem Protein starker Schaden zugefügt wurde.

Ein ausführlicher Vergleich der jeweiligen Ultraschalldüsen wurde im dritten Teil dieser Dissertation durchgeführt. In einer ersten Experimentserie wurde der Einfluss verschiedener

Pumpen auf die Förderhomogenität einer Placebolösung untersucht. Bei dem verwendeten Versuchsaufbau konnten jedoch keine wesentlichen Unterschiede festgestellt werden, unabhängig von den gewählten Bedingungen. Gleiches gilt für den Einfluss der verschiedenen Pumpen auf die resultierenden Partikelgrößenverteilungen. Diese könnten jedoch noch durch das Zusammenfließen einzelner Tropfen nach dem Zerstäuben beeinflusst worden sein. Dennoch erreichten die Ultraschalldüsen trotz Schwankungen in der Förderleistung eine gute Zerstäubungsleistung. Anschließend wurden Zusammenhänge zwischen der Temperatur des Sprühnebels und der Düsenfrequenz untersucht. Höhere Frequenzen und Zerstäubungsleistungen führten zu verstärkter Hitzeabgabe. Die Maximaltemperatur lag bei 80°C für die 120 kHz Düse. Bei vergleichsweise aggressiven Bedingungen (z.B. 120 kHz, 9W) traten deutliche Fluktuationen im Temperatur-Zeit-Profil auf. Da die Temperaturen nicht alleine für den teilweise deutlichen Proteinschaden aus Kapitel 6 verantwortlich sein konnten, wurde das Auftreten von Ultraschall-Kavitation in einer dritten Experimentreihe untersucht. Kavitation führt zur Entstehung freier Radikale, welche Proteine und andere Substanzen oxidieren können. Drei Marker-Lösungen wurden Ultraschalldüsen im Betrieb ausgesetzt und die Zunahme in ihrer Fluoreszenz (TA) oder Absorption (KI, Fe) untersucht. Während die Ergebnisse bei 3W Zerstäubungsleistung noch relativ nah beieinander lagen, wurden die Unterschiede bei höheren Einstellungen ausgeprägter. Die 60 kHz Düse zeigte die geringsten Kavitationseffekte, gefolgt von der 48 kHz und 120 kHz Düse. Letztere führte zu sehr starker Oxidation, die fast mit der eines Ultraschall-Homogenisators vergleichbar war. Die 25 kHz Düse konnte nicht beurteilt werden, da diese bei dem verwendeten experimentellen Aufbau keine kontinuierliche Zerstäubung erreichen konnte. Dies ist in hohem Maße bedauerlich, da dieser Düsentyp die höchste Proteinschädigung in den Experimenten aus Kapitel 6 verursachte. Wie schon bei anderen Versuchen unter aggressiven Zerstäubungsbedingungen nahm auch bei den Kavitationsexperimenten die Standardabweichung bei 9W stark zu. Dies deutet auf eine erhöhte Inhomogenität während des Sprühvorgangs hin.

Im letzten Teil dieser Dissertation wurden verschiedene a-CT/Hilfsstoff-Formulierungen bezüglich ihrer Stabilität untersucht. HSA wurde von diesen Experimenten ausgeschlossen, da es während der vorhergegangen Experimente nicht messbar beeinflusst wurde. a-CT wurde verschiedenen SFD Prozessparametern unterzogen. Bei 60 kHz und 9W konnte a-CT fast vollständig durch die Zugabe von Trehalose, TMD oder TMH stabilisiert werden. Polysorbat 80 konnte den Schaden am Protein nicht merklich reduzieren, was nahelegt, dass Adsorption an die Gas/Wasser-Grenzfläche nur eine untergeordnete Rolle bei den SFD-Experimenten in dieser Arbeit spielte. Folglich scheint der Schaden hauptsächlich durch den Einfrier- und Trocknungsschritt bedingt zu sein, ähnlich wie bei konventioneller Gefriertrocknung. Bei Verwendung aggressiver Bedingungen konnte a-CT nicht mehr durch die klassischen Hilfsstoffe stabilisiert werden. Auswertungen der Sekundär- und Tertiärstruktur sowie der Enzymaktivität zeigten ähnliche, teilweise sogar schlechtere Ergebnisse als die reine Proteinlösung. Deshalb mussten andere Effekte als Einfrieren und Trocknen für den Schaden verantwortlich sein. Durch die Zugabe des Antioxidans Ascorbinsäure konnte die Enzymstabilität verbessert werden. Dies legt nahe, dass Oxidation, die durch Kavitation verursacht wurde, eine Schlüsselrolle für Proteinschädigung unter aggressiven Bedingungen zukommt. Zucker und Polymere stabilisieren hauptsächlich die native Konformation eines Proteins während der Einfrier- und Trocknungsphase. Kavitation könnte demnach die mangelnde Stabilisierung erklären, wenn Zerstäubung bei 120 kHz und 9W durchgeführt wird.

Zusammenfassend war es möglich, mit SFD Mikropartikel mit hoher Proteinbeladung herzustellen. In Bezug auf die Stabilität von Proteinen können keine generellen Schlussfolgerungen gezogen werden, da a-CT und HSA sich während der verschiedenen Prozessschritte gänzlich unterschiedlich verhielten. Unter konservativen Sprühbedingungen zeigten die zusätzlichen Stressfaktoren durch den Zerstäubungsschritt keine messbaren Auswirkungen auf die Proteinstabilität. Dies bedeutet, dass Proteine durch die Zugabe klassischer Kro- und Lyoprotectanten gut stabilisiert werden könnten. Die untersuchten Ultraschalldüsen sind den Zweistoffdüsen in Bezug auf Proteinstabilität nicht unbedingt überlegen. Der Einfluss von Kavitation nimmt unter aggressiveren Bedingungen zu, was zur Destabilisierung von Proteinen führen kann. Auf der anderen Seite bieten Ultraschalldüsen aber die Möglichkeit, Ansätze mit geringem Volumen bei einer niedrigen Förderrate zu versprühen. Zusätzlich erleichtern die verringerten Turbulenzen des flüssigen Stickstoffs beim Versprühen die Versuchsdurchführung erheblich.

Durch die Erstellung eines iPLS Quantifizierungsalgorithmus für FTIR Spektroskopie konnte die Untersuchung der Proteinsekundärstruktur als schnelles und objektives Standardanalysenverfahren integriert werden. Obwohl die Methode weniger sensitiv ist als z.B. die Enzymaktivitätsbestimmung, liefert sie dennoch präzise Informationen bezüglich Proteinstruktur und Proteinstabilität. Eine Übertragung des Algorithmus auf feste Proben würde es ermöglichen, die Sprühgefriertrocknung durch alle Prozessschritte hindurch zu untersuchen. In Bezug auf Kavitation könnte sich eine Weiterentwicklung des Versuchsaufbaus als wertvoll erweisen. Ideal wäre die Messung der in-situ generierten freien Radikale aus einem standardisierten Sprühgefriertrocknungsaufbau heraus. Dadurch könnten die Daten aus einem repräsentativeren Sichtwinkel bestimmt werden. Zusätzlich würde ein Versuchsdesign, das in der Lage ist die 25 kHz Düse zu untersuchen, weitere Erkenntnisse über den Zerstäubungsvorgang ermöglichen. Eine

Untersuchung der Schwankungen bezüglich Temperatur und oxidativem Stress, besonders unter anspruchsvollen Prozessbedingungen, könnte außerdem ein Ansatzpunkt sein, um potentielle Stressfaktoren während der Sprühgefriertrocknung zu verstehen. Abschließend scheint auch eine Untersuchung des Stabilisierungspotentials von Antioxidantien oder Mischungen aus Antioxidantien und klassischen Hilfsstoffen vielversprechend. Diese Formulierungen könnten am Meisten Nutzen bringen, da Proteinschäden während der Sprühgefriertrocknung unter aggressiven Bedingungen höchstwahrscheinlich sowohl von chemischen als auch von physikalischen Instabilitäten verursacht werden. Durch diese Verbesserungen könnte in zukünftigen Arbeiten das Verständnis dieser komplexen Herstellungsweise erweitert werden.

11. References

[Abdul-Fattah et al. 2007] Abdul-Fattah, A. M., Kalonia, D. S. and Pikal, M. J. (2007). "The challenge of drying method selection for protein pharmaceuticals: Product quality implications." J Pharm Sci 96(8): 1886-916.

[Abdul-Fattah et al. 2008] Abdul-Fattah, A. M., Lechuga-Ballesteros, D., Kalonia, D. S., et al. (2008). "The impact of drying method and formulation on the physical properties and stability of methionyl human growth hormone in the amorphous solid state." J Pharm Sci 97(1): 163-84.

[Allison et al. 1999] Allison, S. D., Chang, B., Randolph, T. W., et al. (1999). "Hydrogen bonding between sugar and protein is responsible for inhibition of dehydration-induced protein unfolding." Arch Biochem Biophys 365(2): 289-98.

[Allison et al. 1998] Allison, S. D., Randolph, T. W., Manning, M. C., et al. (1998). "Effects of drying methods and additives on structure and function of actin: mechanisms of dehydration-induced damage and its inhibition." Arch Biochem Biophys 358(1): 171-81.

[Anderle et al. 1987] Anderle, G. and Mendelsohn, R. (1987). "Thermal denaturation of globular proteins. Fourier transform-infrared studies of the amide III spectral region." Biophys J 52(1): 69-74.

[Arakawa et al. 1991] Arakawa, T., Kita, Y. and Carpenter, J. F. (1991). "Protein--solvent interactions in pharmaceutical formulations." Pharm Res 8(3): 285-91.

[Arrondo et al. 1993] Arrondo, J. L., Muga, A., Castresana, J., et al. (1993). "Quantitative studies of the structure of proteins in solution by Fourier-transform infrared spectroscopy." Prog Biophys Mol Biol 59(1): 23-56.

[Baello et al. 2000] Baello, B. I., Pancoska, P. and Keiderling, T. A. (2000). "Enhanced prediction accuracy of protein secondary structure using hydrogen exchange Fourier transform infrared spectroscopy." Anal Biochem 280(1): 46-57.

[Barone 1992] Barone, G. (1992). "DSC studies on the denaturation and aggregation of serum albumins." Thermocimica Acta 199: 197-205.

[Barth et al. 2002] Barth, A. and Zscherp, C. (2002). "What vibrations tell us about proteins." Q Rev Biophys 35(4): 369-430.

[Berger 1998] Berger, H. (1998). Ultrasonic liquid atomization. New York, PartridgeHill Publishers.

[Berman et al. 2000] Berman, H. M., Westbrook, J., Feng, Z., et al. (2000). "The Protein Data Bank." Nucleic Acids Res 28(1): 235-42.

[Burkoth et al. 1999] Burkoth, T. L., Bellhouse, B. J., Hewson, G., et al. (1999). "Transdermal and transmucosal powdered drug delivery." Crit Rev Ther Drug Carrier Syst 16(4): 331-84.

[Carpenter et al. 1998] Carpenter, J. F., Prestrelski, S. J. and Dong, A. (1998). "Application of infrared spectroscopy to development of stable lyophilized protein formulations." Eur J Pharm Biopharm 45(3): 231-8.

[Chalmers et al. 2001] Chalmers, J. and Griffith, P. (2001). Handbook of vibrational spectroscopy. Chichester, John Wiley & Sons.

[Chang et al. 2005] Chang, L. L., Shepherd, D., Sun, J., et al. (2005). "Mechanism of protein stabilization by sugars during freeze-drying and storage: native structure preservation, specific interaction, and/or immobilization in a glassy matrix?" J Pharm Sci 94(7): 1427-44.

[Chen et al. 1998] Chen, Y. and Barkley, M. D. (1998). "Toward understanding tryptophan fluorescence in proteins." Biochemistry 37(28): 9976-82.

[Chi et al. 2003] Chi, E. Y., Krishnan, S., Randolph, T. W., et al. (2003). "Physical stability of proteins in aqueous solution: mechanism and driving forces in nonnative protein aggregation." Pharm Res 20(9): 1325-36.

[Chittur 1998] Chittur, K. K. (1998). "FTIR/ATR for protein adsorption to biomaterial surfaces." Biomaterials 19(4-5): 357-69.

[Chothia et al. 1990] Chothia, C. and Finkelstein, A. V. (1990). "The classification and origins of protein folding patterns." Annu Rev Biochem 59: 1007-39.

[Corey et al. 1951] Corey, R. B. and Pauling, L. (1951). "The pleated sheet, a new layer configuration of polypeptide chains." Proc Natl Acad Sci U S A 37(5): 251-6.

[Costantino et al. 1998] Costantino, H. R., Andya, J. D., Nguyen, P. A., et al. (1998). "Effect of mannitol crystallization on the stability and aerosol performance of a spray-dried pharmaceutical protein, recombinant humanized anti-IgE monoclonal antibody." J Pharm Sci 87(11): 1406-11.

[Costantino et al. 1998] Costantino, H. R., Carrasquillo, K. G., Cordero, R. A., et al. (1998). "Effect of excipients on the stability and structure of lyophilized recombinant human growth hormone." J Pharm Sci 87(11): 1412-20.

[Costantino et al. 2000] Costantino, H. R., Firouzabadian, L., Hogeland, K., et al. (2000). "Protein spray-freeze drying. Effect of atomization conditions on particle size and stability." Pharm Res 17(11): 1374-83.

[Costantino et al. 2002] Costantino, H. R., Firouzabadian, L., Wu, C., et al. (2002). "Protein spray freeze drying. 2. Effect of formulation variables on particle size and stability." J Pharm Sci 91(2): 388-95.

[Costantino et al. 1995] Costantino, H. R., Griebenow, K., Mishra, P., et al. (1995). "Fourier-transform infrared spectroscopic investigation of protein stability in the lyophilized form." Biochim Biophys Acta 1253(1): 69-74.

[Costantino et al. 2004] Costantino, H. R., Pikal, M. J. and American Association of Pharmaceutical Scientists. (2004). Lyophilization of biopharmaceuticals. Arlington, VA, AAPS Press.

[Desie et al. 1986] Desie, G., Boens, N. and De Schryver, F. C. (1986). "Study of the time-resolved tryptophan fluorescence of crystalline alpha-chymotrypsin." Biochemistry 25(25): 8301-8.

[Dong et al. 1995] Dong, A., Prestrelski, S. J., Allison, S. D., et al. (1995). "Infrared spectroscopic studies of lyophilization- and temperature-induced protein aggregation." J Pharm Sci 84(4): 415-24.

[Dousseau et al. 1990] Dousseau, F. and Pezolet, M. (1990). "Determination of the secondary structure content of proteins in aqueous solutions from their amide I and amide II infrared bands. Comparison between classical and partial least-squares methods." Biochemistry 29(37): 8771-9.

[Dudzinski et al. 2008] Dudzinski, D. M. and Kesselheim, A. S. (2008). "Scientific and legal viability of follow-on protein drugs." N Engl J Med 358(8): 843-9.

[Elliott et al. 1950] Elliott, A. and Ambrose, E. J. (1950). "Structure of synthetic polypeptides." Nature 165(4206): 921-2.

[Engelberg et al. 2009] Engelberg, A. B., Kesselheim, A. S. and Avorn, J. (2009). "Balancing Innovation, Access, and Profits -- Market Exclusivity for Biologics." N Engl J Med.

[Engstrom et al. 2007] Engstrom, J. D., Simpson, D. T., Cloonan, C., et al. (2007). "Stable high surface area lactate dehydrogenase particles produced by spray freezing into liquid nitrogen." Eur J Pharm Biopharm 65(2): 163-74.

[Engstrom et al. 2008] Engstrom, J. D., Simpson, D. T., Lai, E. S., et al. (2008). "Morphology of protein particles produced by spray freezing of concentrated solutions." Eur J Pharm Biopharm 65(2): 149-62.

[Forato et al. 1998] Forato, L. A., Bernardes-Filho, R. and Colnago, L. A. (1998). "Protein structure in KBr pellets by infrared spectroscopy." Anal Biochem 259(1): 136-41.

[Frey et al. 1994] Frey, P. A., Whitt, S. A. and Tobin, J. B. (1994). "A low-barrier hydrogen bond in the catalytic triad of serine proteases." Science 264(5167): 1927-30.

[Gelamo et al. 2000] Gelamo, E. L. and Tabak, M. (2000). "Spectroscopic studies on the interaction of bovine (BSA) and human (HSA) serum albumins with ionic surfactants." Spectrochim Acta A Mol Biomol Spectrosc 56A(11): 2255-71.

[Gieseler et al. 2009] Gieseler, H. and Lee, G. (2009). "Gravimetric measurement of momentary drying rate of spray freeze-dried powders in vials." J Pharm Sci 98(9): 3447-55.

[Goodman 2009] Goodman, M. (2009). "Market watch: Sales of biologics to show robust growth through to 2013." Nat Rev Drug Discov 8(11): 837.

[Graumann et al. 2006] Graumann, K. and Premstaller, A. (2006). "Manufacturing of recombinant therapeutic proteins in microbial systems." Biotechnol J 1(2): 164-86.

[Guo 2006] Guo, J. (2006). "Stability of Helix-Rich Proteins at High Concentrations." Biochemistry 45(28): 8686-96.

[Haris et al. 1992] Haris, P. I. and Chapman, D. (1992). "Does Fourier-transform infrared spectroscopy provide useful information on protein structures?" Trends Biochem Sci 17(9): 328-33.

[Haris et al. 1990] Haris, P. I., Chapman, D., Harrison, R. A., et al. (1990). "Conformational transition between native and reactive center cleaved forms of alpha 1-antitrypsin by Fourier transform infrared spectroscopy and small-angle neutron scattering." Biochemistry 29(6): 1377-80.

[Hedin et al. 1982] Hedin, H. and Richter, W. (1982). "Pathomechanisms of dextran-induced anaphylactoid/anaphylactic reactions in man." Int Arch Allergy Appl Immunol 68(2): 122-6.

[Hottot et al. 2007] Hottot, A., Vessot, S. and Andrieu, J. (2007). "Freeze drying of pharmaceuticals in vials: Influence of freezing protocol and sample configuration on ice morphology and freeze-dried cake texture." Chemical Engineering and Processing 46(7): 666-674.

[Hu et al. 2004] Hu, J., Johnston, K. P. and Williams, R. O., 3rd (2004). "Nanoparticle engineering processes for enhancing the dissolution rates of poorly water soluble drugs." Drug Dev Ind Pharm 30(3): 233-45.

[Hu et al. 2002] Hu, J., Rogers, T. L., Brown, J., et al. (2002). "Improvement of dissolution rates of poorly water soluble APIs using novel spray freezing into liquid technology." Pharm Res 19(9): 1278-84.

[Izutsu et al. 2004] Izutsu, K., Aoyagi, N. and Kojima, S. (2004). "Protection of protein secondary structure by saccharides of different molecular weights during freeze-drying." Chem Pharm Bull (Tokyo) 52(2): 199-203.

[Jackson et al. 1995] Jackson, M. and Mantsch, H. H. (1995). "The use and misuse of FTIR spectroscopy in the determination of protein structure." Crit Rev Biochem Mol Biol 30(2): 95-120.

[Johnson et al. 2002] Johnson, R. E., Kirchhoff, C. F. and Gaud, H. T. (2002). "Mannitol-sucrose mixtures--versatile formulations for protein lyophilization." J Pharm Sci 91(4): 914-22.

[Kalnin et al. 1990] Kalnin, N. N., Baikalov, I. A. and Venyaminov, S. (1990). "Quantitative IR spectrophotometry of peptide compounds in water (H2O) solutions. III. Estimation of the protein secondary structure." Biopolymers 30(13-14): 1273-80.

[Kaushik et al. 2003] Kaushik, J. K. and Bhat, R. (2003). "Why is trehalose an exceptional protein stabilizer? An analysis of the thermal stability of proteins in the presence of the compatible osmolyte trehalose." J Biol Chem 278(29): 26458-65.

[Kendall et al. 2004] Kendall, M., Mitchell, T. and Wrighton-Smith, P. (2004). "Intradermal ballistic delivery of micro-particles into excised human skin for pharmaceutical applications." J Biomech 37(11): 1733-41.

[Kendrick et al. 1996] Kendrick, B. S., Dong, A., Allison, S. D., et al. (1996). "Quantitation of the area of overlap between second-derivative amide I infrared spectra to determine the structural similarity of a protein in different states." J Pharm Sci 85(2): 155-8.

[Koda et al. 2003] Koda, S., Kimura, T., Kondo, T., et al. (2003). "A standard method to calibrate sonochemical efficiency of an individual reaction system." Ultrason Sonochem 10(3): 149-56.

[KSB 2009] KSB (2009). "Microchem - Regelbare Pumpe für Kleinstfördermengen" Retrieved 12.10.2009, from www.ksb.de.

[Kumar et al. 2005] Kumar, V., Sharma, V. K. and Kalonia, D. S. (2005). "Second derivative tryptophan fluorescence spectroscopy as a tool to characterize partially unfolded intermediates of proteins." Int J Pharm 294(1-2): 193-9.

[Lakowicz 2006] Lakowicz, J. (2006). Principles of fluorescence spectroscopy. New York, Springer.

[Lee et al. 1990] Lee, D. C., Haris, P. I., Chapman, D., et al. (1990). "Determination of protein secondary structure using factor analysis of infrared spectra." Biochemistry 29(39): 9185-93.

[Lees et al. 2006] Lees, J. G., Miles, A. J., Wien, F., et al. (2006). "A reference database for circular dichroism spectroscopy covering fold and secondary structure space." Bioinformatics 22(16): 1955-62.

[Leuenberger 1987] Leuenberger, H. (1987). Process of drying a particulate material and apparatus for implementing the process. US patent. 4,608,764: 15p.

[Leuenberger 2002] Leuenberger, H. (2002). "Spray freeze-drying – the process of choice for low water soluble drugs?" Journal of Nanoparticle Research 4(1-2): 111-119.

[Levitt et al. 1977] Levitt, M. and Greer, J. (1977). "Automatic identification of secondary structure in globular proteins." J Mol Biol 114(2): 181-239.

[Lin et al. 2000] Lin, J. J., Meyer, J. D., Carpenter, J. F., et al. (2000). "Stability of human serum albumin during bioprocessing: denaturation and aggregation during processing of albumin paste." Pharm Res 17(4): 391-6.

[Linde 2008] Linde (2008). "Data sheet" Retrieved 2009-11-24, from http://www.linde-gase.de/produkte/industriegase/industriegase.html.

[Lorber 1987] Lorber, A. (1987). "A theoretical foundation for the PLS algorithm." Journal of Chemometrics 1: 19-31.

[Luthra et al. 2007] Luthra, S., Obert, J. P., Kalonia, D. S., et al. (2007). "Impact of critical process and formulation parameters affecting in-process stability of lactate dehydrogenase during the secondary drying stage of lyophilization: A mini freeze dryer study." J Pharm Sci.

[Maa 2001] Maa, Y. F. (2001). Method of spray freeze drying proteins for pharmaceutical administration. United States Patent. USA, Genentech, Inc. US 6,284,282: 26.

[Maa et al. 2004] Maa, Y. F., Ameri, M., Shu, C., et al. (2004). "Influenza vaccine powder formulation development: spray-freeze-drying and stability evaluation." J Pharm Sci 93(7): 1912-23.

[Maa et al. 1998] Maa, Y. F., Nguyen, P. A. and Hsu, S. W. (1998). "Spray-drying of air-liquid interface sensitive recombinant human growth hormone." J Pharm Sci 87(2): 152-9.

[Maa et al. 1999] Maa, Y. F., Nguyen, P. A., Sweeney, T., et al. (1999). "Protein inhalation powders: spray drying vs spray freeze drying." Pharm Res 16(2): 249-54.

[Maa et al. 2000] Maa, Y. F. and Prestrelski, S. J. (2000). "Biopharmaceutical powders: particle formation and formulation considerations." Curr Pharm Biotechnol 1(3): 283-302.

[Maa et al. 2003] Maa, Y. F., Zhao, L., Payne, L. G., et al. (2003). "Stabilization of alum-adjuvanted vaccine dry powder formulations: mechanism and application." J Pharm Sci 92(2): 319-32.

[Makrides 1996] Makrides, S. C. (1996). "Strategies for achieving high-level expression of genes in Escherichia coli." Microbiol Rev 60(3): 512-38.

[Malik et al. 2007] Malik, D. K., Baboota, S., Ahuja, A., et al. (2007). "Recent advances in protein and peptide drug delivery systems." Curr Drug Deliv 4(2): 141-51.

[Manning 1989] Manning, M. C. (1989). "Underlying assumptions in the estimation of secondary structure content in proteins by circular dichroism spectroscopy--a critical review." J Pharm Biomed Anal 7(10): 1103-19.

[Manning et al. 1989] Manning, M. C., Patel, K. and Borchardt, R. T. (1989). "Stability of protein pharmaceuticals." Pharm Res 6(11): 903-18.

[Masters 1991] Masters, K. (1991). Spray-Drying Handbook. New York, Wiley & Sons.

[Mauerer 2006] Mauerer, A. (2006). Secondary structural changes of spray dried proteins with fourier transform infrared spectroscopy. Division of pharmaceutics. Erlangen, FAU Erlangen - Nuremberg: 189.

[Maury et al. 2005] Maury, M., Murphy, K., Kumar, S., et al. (2005). "Effects of process variables on the powder yield of spray-dried trehalose on a laboratory spray-dryer." Eur J Pharm Biopharm 59(3): 565-73.

[McLean et al. 1988] McLean, J. R. and Mortimer, A. J. (1988). "A cavitation and free radical dosimeter for ultrasound." Ultrasound Med Biol 14(1): 59-64.

[Meister et al. 2008] Meister, E. and Gieseler, H. (2008). "Freeze-dry microscopy of protein/sugar mixtures: Drying behavior, interpretation of collapse temperatures and a comparison to corresponding glass transition Data." J Pharm Sci.

[Minton 1997] Minton, A. P. (1997). "Influence of excluded volume upon macromolecular structure and associations in 'crowded' media." Curr Opin Biotechnol 8(1): 65-9.

[Minton 2000] Minton, A. P. (2000). "Implications of macromolecular crowding for protein assembly." Curr Opin Struct Biol 10(1): 34-9.

[Moelbert et al. 2004] Moelbert, S., Normand, B. and De Los Rios, P. (2004). "Kosmotropes and chaotropes: modelling preferential exclusion, binding and aggregate stability." Biophys Chem 112(1): 45-57.

[Moran et al. 1977] Moran, E. C., Chou, P. Y. and Fasman, G. D. (1977). "Conformational transitions of glucagon in solution: the alpha to beta transition." Biochem Biophys Res Commun 77(4): 1300-6.

[Muzammil et al. 1999] Muzammil, S., Kumar, Y. and Tayyab, S. (1999). "Molten globule-like state of human serum albumin at low pH." Eur J Biochem 266(1): 26-32.

[Navea et al. 2005] Navea, S., Tauler, R. and de Juan, A. (2005). "Application of the local regression method interval partial least-squares to the elucidation of protein secondary structure." Anal Biochem 336(2): 231-42.

[Onoue et al. 2006] Onoue, S., Iwasa, S., Kojima, T., et al. (2006). "Structural transition of glucagon in the concentrated solution observed by electrophoretic and spectroscopic techniques." J Chromatogr A 1109(2): 167-73.

[Onoue et al. 2004] Onoue, S., Ohshima, K., Debari, K., et al. (2004). "Mishandling of the therapeutic peptide glucagon generates cytotoxic amyloidogenic fibrils." Pharm Res 21(7): 1274-83.

[Pauling et al. 1951] Pauling, L. and Corey, R. B. (1951). "Configuration of polypeptide chains." Nature 168(4274): 550-1.

[Pikal-Cleland et al. 2001] Pikal-Cleland, K. A. and Carpenter, J. F. (2001). "Lyophilization-induced protein denaturation in phosphate buffer systems: monomeric and tetrameric beta-galactosidase." J Pharm Sci 90(9): 1255-68.

[Porter 1994] Porter, M. R. (1994). Handbook of surfactants. Glasgow, Springer Netherlands.

[Prestrelski et al. 1993] Prestrelski, S. J., Arakawa, T. and Carpenter, J. F. (1993). "Separation of freezing- and drying-induced denaturation of lyophilized proteins using stress-specific stabilization. II. Structural studies using infrared spectroscopy." Arch Biochem Biophys 303(2): 465-73.

[Prestrelski et al. 1993] Prestrelski, S. J., Tedeschi, N., Arakawa, T., et al. (1993). "Dehydration-induced conformational transitions in proteins and their inhibition by stabilizers." Biophys J 65(2): 661-71.

[Purvis et al. 2006] Purvis, T., Vaughn, J. M., Rogers, T. L., et al. (2006). "Cryogenic liquids, nanoparticles, and microencapsulation." Int J Pharm 324(1): 43-50.

[Rahmelow et al. 1996] Rahmelow, K. and Hubner, W. (1996). "Secondary structure determination of proteins in aqueous solution by infrared spectroscopy: a comparison of multivariate data analysis methods." Anal Biochem 241(1): 5-13.

[Rambhatla et al. 2003] Rambhatla, S. and Pikal, M. J. (2003). "Heat and mass transfer scale-up issues during freeze-drying, I: atypical radiation and the edge vial effect." AAPS PharmSciTech 4(2): E14.

[Rey et al. 2004] Rey, L. and May, J., Eds. (2004). Freeze-Drying / Lyophilization of Pharmaceutical and Biological Products, Informa Healthcare.

[Riesz et al. 1992] Riesz, P. and Kondo, T. (1992). "Free radical formation induced by ultrasound and its biological implications." Free Radic Biol Med 13(3): 247-70.

[Rochelle 2005] Rochelle, C. (2005). Spray-freeze-dried protein powders for needle-free injection. Department of pharmaceutics. Erlangen, FAU Erlangen-Nürnberg. PhD Thesis: 153p.

[Rochelle et al. 2007] Rochelle, C. and Lee, G. (2007). "Dextran or hydroxyethyl starch in spray-freeze-dried trehalose/mannitol microparticles intended as ballistic particulate carriers for proteins." J Pharm Sci 96(9): 2296-309.

[Rogers et al. 2003] Rogers, T. L., Johnston, K. P. and Williams, R. O., 3rd (2003). "Physical stability of micronized powders produced by spray-freezing into liquid (SFL) to enhance the dissolution of an insoluble drug." Pharm Dev Technol 8(2): 187-97.

[Rogers et al. 2002] Rogers, T. L., Nelsen, A. C., Hu, J., et al. (2002). "A novel particle engineering technology to enhance dissolution of poorly water soluble drugs: spray-freezing into liquid." Eur J Pharm Biopharm 54(3): 271-80.

[Roswell 2008] Roswell, L., Ed. (2008). Protein Conformation: New Research. New York, Nova Science Pub Inc.

[Rupley et al. 1991] Rupley, J. A. and Careri, G. (1991). "Protein hydration and function." Adv Protein Chem 41: 37-172.

[Sarver et al. 1991] Sarver, R. W., Jr. and Krueger, W. C. (1991). "Protein secondary structure from Fourier transform infrared spectroscopy: a data base analysis." Anal Biochem 194(1): 89-100.

[Scharnagl et al. 2005] Scharnagl, C., Reif, M. and Friedrich, J. (2005). "Stability of proteins: temperature, pressure and the role of the solvent." Biochim Biophys Acta 1749(2): 187-213.

[Schiffter 2007] Schiffter, H. (2007). High concentrated protein particles for needle-free ballistic powder delivery prepared via spray-freeze-drying. AAPS Annual Meeting, 2007.

[Schneid et al. 2008] Schneid, S. C., Gieseler, H., Kessler, W. J., et al. (2008). "Non-invasive product temperature determination during primary drying using tunable diode laser absorption spectroscopy." J Pharm Sci.

[Shah et al. 1999] Shah, Y. T. and Pandit, A. B. (1999). Cavitation reaction engineering. New York, Kluwer Academic / Plenum Publishers.

[Shamblin et al. 2000] Shamblin, S. L., Hancock, B. C., Dupuis, Y., et al. (2000). "Interpretation of relaxation time constants for amorphous pharmaceutical systems." J Pharm Sci 89(3): 417-27.

[Siekmeier et al. 2008] Siekmeier, R. and Scheuch, G. (2008). "Inhaled insulin--does it become reality?" J Physiol Pharmacol 59 Suppl 6: 81-113.

[Sigma-Aldrich 2009] Sigma-Aldrich (2009). "Enzyme explorer - chymotrypsin" Retrieved 29.10.2009, from http://www.sigmaaldrich.com/life-science/metabolomics/enzyme-explorer/analytical-enzymes/chymotrypsin.html.

[Sonner 2002] Sonner, C. (2002). Protein-loaded powders by spray freeze drying. Division of pharmaceutics. Erlangen, FAU Erlangen - Nuremberg. PhD Thesis: 150p.

[Sonner et al. 2002] Sonner, C., Maa, Y. F. and Lee, G. (2002). "Spray-freeze-drying for protein powder preparation: particle characterization and a case study with trypsinogen stability." J Pharm Sci 91(10): 2122-39.

[Sono-Tek 2005] Sono-Tek (2005). Ultrasonic spray nozzle systems. New York: 1-16.

[Sono-Tek 2009] Sono-Tek (2009). "Nozzle Technology" Retrieved 20.09.2009, from http://www.sono-tek.com/electronics/page/3/1.

[Sponer 1990] Sponer, J. (1990). "Dependence of the cavitation threshold on the ultrasonic frequency." Czech. J. Phys. 40: 1123-1132.

[Sreerama et al. 1999] Sreerama, N., Venyaminov, S. Y. and Woody, R. W. (1999). "Estimation of the number of alpha-helical and beta-strand segments in proteins using circular dichroism spectroscopy." Protein Sci 8(2): 370-80.

[Sreerama et al. 2000] Sreerama, N. and Woody, R. W. (2000). "Estimation of protein secondary structure from circular dichroism spectra: comparison of CONTIN, SELCON, and CDSSTR methods with an expanded reference set." Anal Biochem 287(2): 252-60.

[Stryer et al. 2008] Stryer, L., Berg, J. and Tymoczko, J. (2008). Biochemstry. New York, W. H. Freeman.

[Susi et al. 1985] Susi, H., Byler, D. M. and Purcell, J. M. (1985). "Estimation of beta-structure content of proteins by means of deconvolved FTIR spectra." J Biochem Biophys Methods 11(4-5): 235-40.

[Tang et al. 2004] Tang, X. and Pikal, M. J. (2004). "Design of freeze-drying processes for pharmaceuticals: practical advice." Pharm Res 21(2): 191-200.

[Timasheff 2002] Timasheff, S. N. (2002). "Protein hydration, thermodynamic binding, and preferential hydration." Biochemistry 41(46): 13473-82.

[Trewhella et al. 1989] Trewhella, J., Liddle, W. K., Heidorn, D. B., et al. (1989). "Calmodulin and troponin C structures studied by Fourier transform infrared spectroscopy: effects of Ca2+ and Mg2+ binding." Biochemistry 28(3): 1294-301.

[van de Weert et al. 2000] van de Weert, M., Hennink, W. E. and Jiskoot, W. (2000). "Protein instability in poly(lactic-co-glycolic acid) microparticles." Pharm Res 17(10): 1159-67.

[van der Weert et al. 2005] van der Weert, M., Hering, J. and Haris, P. (2005). Methods for Structural Analysis of Protein Pharmaceuticals. Biotechnology: Pharmaceutical Aspects. In: Jiskoot, W.et al (Eds.). New York, AAPS Press: 131-166.

[van Drooge et al. 2005] van Drooge, D. J., Hinrichs, W. L., Dickhoff, B. H., et al. (2005). "Spray freeze drying to produce a stable Delta(9)-tetrahydrocannabinol containing inulin-based solid dispersion powder suitable for inhalation." Eur J Pharm Sci 26(2): 231-40.

[Vermeer et al. 2000] Vermeer, A. W. and Norde, W. (2000). "The thermal stability of immunoglobulin: unfolding and aggregation of a multi-domain protein." Biophys J 78(1): 394-404.

[Vivian et al. 2001] Vivian, J. T. and Callis, P. R. (2001). "Mechanisms of tryptophan fluorescence shifts in proteins." Biophys J 80(5): 2093-109.

[Vonhoff 2007] Vonhoff, S. (2007). Investigation of protein process stability during spray-freeze-drying (SFD) using FTIR and fluorescence spectroscopy. AAPS annual meeting, San Diego.

[Vonhoff 2008] Vonhoff, S. (2008). FTIR in der Praxis. Gerfriertrocknung in der Praxis - Das Erlangen Seminar, Erlangen, Germany.

[Vonhoff 2009] Vonhoff, S. (2009). "The determination of structural changes of biopharmaceuticals during Freeze-Drying using Fourier Transform Infrared Spectroscopy." European Pharmaceutical Review(2): 57-64.

[Vonhoff et al. 2009] Vonhoff, S., Condliffe, J. and Schiffter, H. (2009). "Implementation of an FTIR calibration curve for fast and objective determination of changes in protein secondary structure during formulation development." J Pharm Biomed Anal 51(1): 39-45.

[Walsh 2001] Walsh, G. (2001). Proteins: Biotechnology and Biochemistry. Hoboken, Wiley & Sons.

[Wan et al. 1974] Wan, L. S. and Lee, P. F. (1974). "CMC of polysorbates." J Pharm Sci 63(1): 136-7.

[Wang et al. 2004] Wang, J., Chua, K. M. and Wang, C. H. (2004). "Stabilization and encapsulation of human immunoglobulin G into biodegradable microspheres." J Colloid Interface Sci 271(1): 92-101.

[Wang et al. 2005] Wang, S. L., Lin, S. Y., Li, M. J., et al. (2005). "Temperature effect on the structural stability, similarity, and reversibility of human serum albumin in different states." Biophys Chem 114(2-3): 205-12.

[Wang 1999] Wang, W. (1999). "Instability, stabilization, and formulation of liquid protein pharmaceuticals." Int J Pharm 185(2): 129-88.

[Wang 2000] Wang, W. (2000). "Lyophilization and development of solid protein pharmaceuticals." Int J Pharm 203(1-2): 1-60.

[Wang 2005] Wang, W. (2005). "Protein aggregation and its inhibition in biopharmaceutics." Int J Pharm 289(1-2): 1-30.

[Wang 1988] Wang, Y. (1988). "Parenteral Formulations of Proteins and Peptides: Stability and Stabilizers." Journal of Parenteral Science and Technology 42(Supplement 2): S4-S26.

[Wang et al. 2008] Wang, Y., Boysen, R. I., Wood, B. R., et al. (2008). "Determination of the secondary structure of proteins in different environments by FTIR-ATR spectroscopy and PLS regression." Biopolymers 89(11): 895-905.

[Wang et al. 2006] Wang, Z. L., Finlay, W. H., Peppler, M. S., et al. (2006). "Powder formation by atmospheric spray-freeze-drying." Powder Technology 170: 45-52.

[Webb et al. 2002] Webb, S. D., Golledge, S. L., Cleland, J. L., et al. (2002). "Surface adsorption of recombinant human interferon-gamma in lyophilized and spray-lyophilized formulations." J Pharm Sci 91(6): 1474-87.

[Whitmore et al. 2008] Whitmore, L. and Wallace, B. A. (2008). "Protein secondary structure analyses from circular dichroism spectroscopy: methods and reference databases." Biopolymers 89(5): 392-400.

[Wi et al. 1998] Wi, S., Pancoska, P. and Keiderling, T. A. (1998). "Predictions of protein secondary structures using factor analysis on Fourier transform infrared spectra: effect of Fourier self-deconvolution of the amide I and amide II bands." Biospectroscopy 4(2): 93-106.

[Williams 2005] Williams, R. O., 3rd (2005). Process for production of nanoparticles and microparticles by spray freezing into liquid. United States Patent. USA, Bord of regents, University of Texas. 6,862,890: 12.

[Wirnt 1974] Wirnt, R. (1974). Methods of Enzymatic Analysis. New York, Academic Press Inc.

[Wu 2001] Wu, Y. (2001). "Two-dimensional infrared spectroscopy and principal component analysis studies of the secondary structure and kinetics of hydrogen-deuterium exchange of human serum albumin." Journal of Physical Chemistry B 105(26): 6251-6259.

[Yu et al. 2004] Yu, Z., Garcia, A. S., Johnston, K. P., et al. (2004). "Spray freezing into liquid nitrogen for highly stable protein nanostructured microparticles." Eur J Pharm Biopharm 58(3): 529-37.

[Yu et al. 2006] Yu, Z., Johnston, K. P. and Williams, R. O., 3rd (2006). "Spray freezing into liquid versus spray-freeze drying: influence of atomization on protein aggregation and biological activity." Eur J Pharm Sci 27(1): 9-18.

[Yu et al. 2002] Yu, Z., Rogers, T. L., Hu, J., et al. (2002). "Preparation and characterization of microparticles containing peptide produced by a novel process: spray freezing into liquid." Eur J Pharm Biopharm 54(2): 221-8.

[Zhou et al. 1997] Zhou, T. and Rosen, B. P. (1997). "Tryptophan fluorescence reports nucleotide-induced conformational changes in a domain of the ArsA ATPase." J Biol Chem 272(32): 19731-7.

[Ziegler 2006] Ziegler, A. S. (2006). "Inactivation Effects on Proteins in a Needle-Free Vaccine Injector." Eng. Life Sci. 6(4): 384-393.

MIX
Papier aus verantwortungsvollen Quellen
Paper from responsible sources
FSC® C105338

Printed by Books on Demand GmbH, Norderstedt / Germany